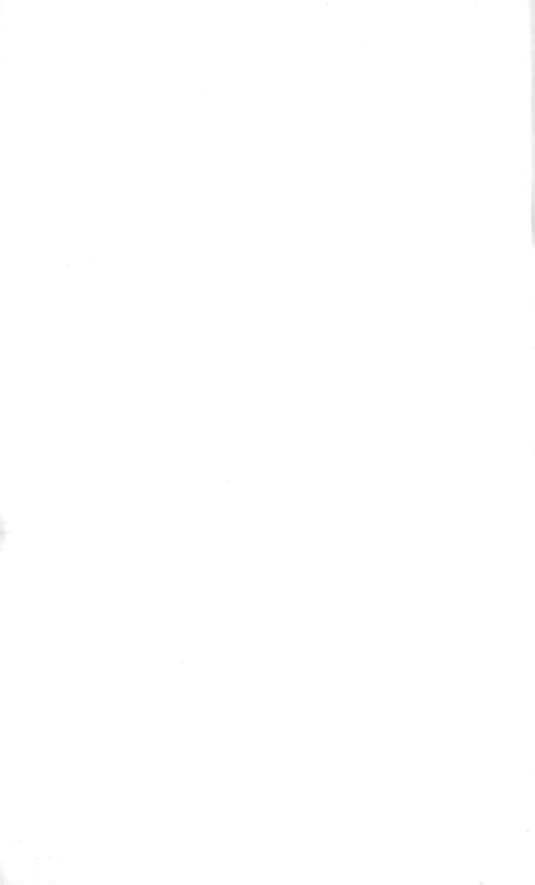

Outcome Measurements in Cardiovascular Medicine

Edited by
Kenneth J. Tuman, M.D.
The Max S. Sadove, M.D. Professor and Vice Chair
Department of Anesthesiology
Rush Medical College
Rush-Presbyterian-St. Luke's Medical Center
Chicago, Illinois

With 10 contributors

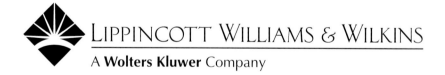

Outcome Measurements in Cardiovascular Medicine

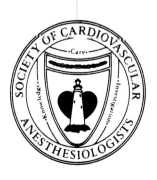

A Society of
Cardiovascular Anesthesiologists
Monograph

Copyright © 1999
SOCIETY OF CARDIOVASCULAR ANESTHESIOLOGISTS

All rights reserved, This book is protected by copyright. No part of this book may be reproduced in any form or by any means, including photocopying, or utilized by any information storage and retrieval system without written permission from the copyright owner.

Accurate indications, adverse reactions, and dosage schedules for drugs are provided in this book, but it is possible that they may change. The reader is urged to review the package information data of the manufacturers of the medications mentioned.

Printed in the United States of America
(ISBN 0-781-72223-3)

99 00 01
1 2 3 4 5 6 7 8 9 10

Publication Committee of the
Society of Cardiovascular Anesthesiologists

Mark Newman, M.D., Chairman
Durham, North Carolina

William Greeley, M.D., Vice-Chairman
Philadelphia, Pennsylvania

Carl Lynch III, M.D., Ph.D.
Charlottesville, Virginia

Thomas J. J. Blanck, M.D.
New York, New York

Peter Slinger, M.D.
Toronto, Ontario, Canada

Brian Cason, M.D.
San Francisco, California

David Larach, M.D., Ph.D.
Owings Mills, Maryland

Michael Urban, M.D.
Greenwich, Connecticut

Preface

Perioperative cardiac morbidity remains the leading cause of death following surgery and anesthesia, and the impact of cardiovascular disease on perioperative outcome is significant because the incidence of cardiovascular disease is high and is increasing as the world population ages. The importance of proper methods for assessing outcome and quality of care is highlighted by the following example. In the 1950's internal mammary artery ligation was popularized as an efficacious treatment for coronary artery disease based on the assumption that this procedure would divert blood flow to the coronary arteries. Increased exercise tolerance and relief of angina pectoris were attributed to this procedure, and its use was not abandoned until a randomized clinical trial demonstrated no difference in outcomes after internal mammary artery ligation compared with sham operations. While this single example should leave little doubt that properly conducted outcomes studies are crucial to validate the effects of disease states and therapy, four decades later we continue to struggle with defining the optimal method for assessing outcomes. Effective strategies to modify perioperative care and reduce risk can only be successfully developed when we have information about baseline outcomes and can then determine if specifically targeted interventions have improved that outcome or another measure of quality of care.

Although a monograph of this size cannot provide exhaustive coverage of all important issues related to outcomes assessment, it represents an attempt to provide a broad overview of several important facets of outcome measurement in cardiovascular medicine. The disciplines of anesthesiology, cardiology, internal medicine and surgery have all contributed to increasing efforts to understand the best methods to obtain and apply outcome data to clinical decision making. The authors contributing to this monograph are leaders in the field of outcomes research and provide broad multidisciplinary perspectives on our current state of knowledge of how to obtain and apply outcome data.

After reading this monograph, it will be apparent that outcomes assessment in cardiovascular medicine is an exceedingly important but still underdeveloped discipline. Perhaps that realization will stimulate those who read this monograph to contribute to the science of outcomes assessment in patients with cardiovascular disease. This remains an important challenge which will require exhausting efforts, but as illustrated in this monograph, will likely yield tangible and substantial benefits for our patients.

Contributors

Karen B. Domino, M.D., M.P.H.
Professor of Anesthesiology
University of Washington
Seattle, Washington

Dennis M. Fisher, M.D.
Professor of Anesthesia and Pediatrics
Department of Anesthesia
University of California
San Francisco, California

Lee A. Fleisher, M.D.
Associate Professor and Chief
Division of Perioperative Health
    Services Research
Joint Appointments in Medicine and
    Health Policy & Management
Johns Hopkins Medical Institutions
Baltimore, Maryland

James G. Jollis, M.D.
Assistant Professor of Medicine
Division of Cardiology
Department of Medicine
Duke University Medical Center
Durham, North Carolina

David A. Lubarsky, M.D.
Professor
Department of Anesthesiology
Duke University Medical Center
Durham, North Carolina

Dennis T. Mangano, Ph.D. M.D.
Director
McSPI Research Group
San Francisco, California

Fredrick K. Orkin, M.D.
Professor of Health Services Research
    and of Anesthesia
Pennsylvania State College of
    Medicine
Anesthesiologist
Milton S. Hershey Medical Center
Pennsylvania State Geisinger Health
    System
Hershey, Pennsylvania

Jeffrey H. Silber, M.D., Ph.D.
Director, Center for Outcomes
    Research
The Children's Hospital of
    Philadelphia
Associate Professor of Pediatrics,
    Anesthesiology, and Health Care
    Systems
The University of Pennsylvania
    School of Medicine and the
    Wharton School
Philadelphia, Pennsylvania

T. Samuel Shomaker, M.D., J.D.
Interim Dean
University of Utah School of
    Medicine
Salt Lake City, Utah

Barbara E. Tardiff, M.D.
Assistant Professor of
  Anesthesiology
Division of Cardiothoracic
  Anesthesia
Department of Anesthesiology
Duke University Medical Center
Durham, North Carolina

Contents

Preface   vii

Contributors   ix

1   1
Using Outcomes Analysis to Assess Quality of Care: Applications for Cardiovascular Surgery
    Jeffrey H. Silber

2   23
How Do We Obtain Outcome Data: Randomized Clinical Trials Versus Observational Data Bases?
    Dennis M. Fisher

3   39
Application of Outcomes Research to Clinical Decision Making in Cardiovascular Medicine
    Fredrick K. Orkin

4   67
The Use of Information Systems and Large Databases in Cardiovascular Medicine
    Barbara E. Tardiff
    James G. Jollis
    David A. Lubarsky

5 — 81
Principles of Outcome Prediction in Patients with Coronary Artery Disease
Lee A. Fleisher

6 — 105
Outcome Studies in Perioperative Medicine: The β-Blockade Trials
Dennis T. Mangano

7 — 125
Practice Guidelines in Cardiovascular Anesthesia
T. Samuel Shomaker

8 — 159
Closed Claims Analysis as a Tool for Outcome Assessment
Karen B. Domino

Index — 173

Jeffrey H. Silber

1 Using Outcomes Analysis to Assess Quality of Care: Applications for Cardiovascular Surgery

Over the past 10 years, the financing and organization of healthcare has undergone great changes. The rise of managed care organizations and capitation contracts have increased the need for valid and reliable quality of care measures. Without reliable quality of care measures, value and efficiency cannot be defined, because cost savings may, in some instances, simply be the result of quality reduction. The measurement of quality is therefore central to any evaluation of healthcare policy.

Initiatives in cardiovascular surgery have, early on, developed models for quality interventions to better define and improve outcomes. Projects such as the New York State coronary artery bypass graft hospital and provider reports[1,2] and the Northern New England Cardiovascular Disease Study Group[3,4] have lead these efforts to improve quality of care. Given the importance of quality assessment and the large impact such studies have on all fields of medicine, it is useful to critically review and evaluate these quality of care initiatives and ask how they can be improved or expanded.

In this chapter, I examine outcome measures, with an emphasis on applications from studies on cardiovascular surgery concerning quality of care. The fundamental properties of the ideal outcome statistic; the concept of failure to rescue, a measure that may help to improve outcomes analyses; the problem of upcoding bias in the two cardiovascular outcomes studies noted above; and recommendations for future outcomes research in cardiovascular surgery follow.

Outcome Measurements, edited by Kenneth Tuman, Lippincott Williams & Wilkins, Baltimore © 1999

THE IDEAL OUTCOME MEASURE

In any outcome study, the most important decision made by the investigators is the selection of the outcome measure. Results often vary according to the outcome measure chosen, so it is essential to have an adequate framework for making such a decision. Table 1–1 lists nine properties of the ideal outcome measure.

The first property of an outcome measure is that it should reflect the quality of care of the hospital or provider. Although obvious and often taken for granted, this property is not achieved in many outcome studies. It may be difficult for an outcome measure to display this property if it is not clear whether the outcome of interest is truly a function of the provider's actions. Indeed, it may be the case that actions across providers are either completely uniform or, if heterogeneous, these actions may be completely inconsequential when assessing outcome—that is, the variability in outcomes may only be a function of patient characteristics. Suppose we choose to look at survival from advanced pancreatic cancer. Because treatment does not influence the course of the disease, ranking providers simply by mortality would not provide insight into quality of care. An outcome measure of quality of care must be a function of provider actions.

Outcomes should be predictable. To develop meaningful measures that compare observed with expected results, one must be able to estimate the expected results with some precision. If outcomes are simply random, leaving no basis for estimating the expected result, then comparison with the observed rate becomes less informative. If, however, one can reasonably estimate the expected frequency of an event, then deviations from the expected frequency may be of interest.

Ideally, an outcome measure should reflect hospital or provider quality without being dependent on correction for severity of illness. If the selected outcome measure did not need severity correction to properly account for differences in patient severity and case mix, then the errors in severity correction commonly associated with adminis-

TABLE 1–1. PROPERTIES OF THE IDEAL OUTCOME MEASURE

Reflects quality of care of the provider
Can be predicted or estimated from a model
Not overly dependent on inadequate severity correction
Has construct validity
Has adequate statistical power
Uniformly defined
Uniformly observed
Uniformly recorded
Inexpensive to measure

trative claims data would not have the adverse consequences commonly associated with inadequate severity correction. An outcome measure that levels the playing field across hospitals without requiring detailed severity adjustments would be very desirable. Of course, no such outcome measure exists, yet severity correction, to a greater or lesser degree, influences various measures. The better outcome measures are those that can "get it right" and level the playing field across hospitals and providers with minimal severity adjustment; i.e., they are robust and stable across different levels of precision in severity adjustment.

Outcome measures should have construct validity.[5] Messick[6] defined construct validity as follows: "Construct validation is a process of marshaling evidence to support the inference that an observed response consistency in test performance has a particular meaning, primarily by appraising the extent to which empirical relationships with other measures, or the lack thereof, are consistent with the meaning." Factors associated with an outcome measure should be plausible and consistent. If a new quality measure fails to be correlated with other factors generally associated with quality, then we must ask whether this new outcome measure does indeed measure quality of care. If the rankings of hospitals based on a new outcome measure are uncorrelated with hospital rankings based on mortality (a traditional outcome measure), then we must ask whether the new hospital quality measure has construct validity and treat the new, uncorrelated measure with some skepticism.

In the case of the complication rate, a commonly used outcome measure, we have seen that reasonable factors thought to improve hospital quality of care are associated with increased complication rates. Higher nurse staffing ratios, teaching status, and high level of technology have all been associated with increased complication rates.[7] Furthermore, as described below, we have seen almost no correlation between hospital complication rates and hospital death rates after severity adjustment. With such poor construct validity, one may question the usefulness of this outcome measure.

At times, seemingly well correlated outcomes may, on further examination, prove to have little or no association. In a study of 74,647 general surgical procedures performed at 142 hospitals, we found that the correlation between hospital rankings of death and complication rates was greatly influenced by the extent of case mix and severity adjustment.[5] Table 1–2 displays four models used to rank hospitals by death and complication rates. A full model refers to adjustment with admission severity score, comorbidity status, emergency status, Diagnosis-Related Groups and procedure groupings, and demographic variables, including age and sex. As information is subtracted from the

TABLE 1–2. CORRELATIONS BETWEEN DEATH (D) AND COMPLICATION (C) RATE RANKINGS IN MODELS WITH SUCCESSIVELY DECREASING INFORMATION ON COVARIATES

Model	Description	C Statistic	C Statistic	Correlation	
				D versus C	95% CI
I	Full	0.92	0.86	0.21	0.04, 0.38
II	Full without severity score	0.90	0.85	0.27	0.09, 0.43
III	Full without severity score; history or emergency status	0.88	0.83	0.35	0.19, 0.53
IV	No model; unadjusted	—	—	0.55	0.38, 0.72

Data taken from Reference 5.

model, the correlation between death and complication measures increases. The best correlation occurs when there is no adjustment, just raw death and complication rates. With no adjustment, the Spearman rank correlation between measures was 0.55; with full adjustment, the correlation between these two outcome measures fell to 0.21. We have shown that the spuriously high correlation is a function of the size of the partial correlations among death, complication, and severity adjustment covariates.[5] Before one can conclude that complication rates are an adequate measure of quality of care, there should be evidence that complication rates are highly correlated with mortality after a thorough adjustment for initial severity of illness. When a correlation between two outcomes measures is present before complete severity adjustment, it may simply reflect the strong correlation between patients' severity of illness and mortality and between patients' severity and complications.

All outcome measures must, in the end, meet certain statistical constraints associated with adequate power. Outcome statistics may differ in their ability to distinguish across providers. The mortality rate may have inadequate power to detect differences across hospitals in conditions in which mortality is low. Table 1–3 provides an example of a power analysis. It assumes that one wants to compare mortality rates between two hospitals of equal size, with a prespecified type I or α error of 5%, at least an interesting difference of 50% (that is, the desired level of detection is the ability to observe at least a 50% increase in mortality), and a desired type II error of 20%, corresponding to a power of 80% (or an 80% chance of detecting at least a 50% difference in death rates).[8,9] As shown in Table 2, 1500 patients per hospital would be required to detect a 50% difference in a death rate as low as 5%. Such numbers may be impractical to obtain or may require grouping of procedures or lengthen-

TABLE 1–3. POWER AND SAMPLE SIZE FOR SPECIFIED DEATH RATES

Death Rate (%)	Sample Size per Hospital
2.5	3194
5	1547
10	725
20	312
30	175
40	107
50	65

Assuming type I error = 5%; type II error 20% (power 80%); least interesting difference 50%; equal numbers of patients at both hospitals.

ing the time period of data collection. Both alternatives may imply less relevant data for policy makers. As a consequence, many investigators have been studying more common outcomes, such as complications.[10-14] However, as discussed later in this chapter, the use of the complication rate is fraught with problems and can easily lead investigators to the wrong conclusions when making comparisons across hospitals.[15]

It is essential that outcomes selected for comparing quality of care across hospitals or providers be uniformly defined. Mortality is generally considered to be uniformly defined, yet differences may arise across studies. For example, in-hospital death versus death 30 days postadmission may lead to differences in outcome rankings (although most studies are reassuring concerning the magnitude of these differences).[16,17] Greater differences in outcomes may occur when comparing interhospital complication rates.

Once definitions of outcomes are made uniform, it is also essential to uniformly observe such outcomes. Different hospitals may have different policies concerning the ascertainment of medical tests, which may influence the rate of observed events and, therefore, the complication rate. An ideal example from cardiovascular surgery is the use of cardiac enzymes after coronary artery bypass surgery as a marker for postbypass infarction. We have observed that some hospitals routinely perform such tests, using a higher threshold for determining a positive result than the threshold used in the emergency department. Other hospitals do not draw post-coronary artery bypass grafting (CABG) enzymes unless clinically indicated. The hospitals that routinely draw enzymes generally have higher rates of post-CABG infarction, yet this does not imply worse quality of care.

It is not enough for an outcome measure to be uniformly defined and observed; it must also be uniformly recorded if claims data are to be used to construct a quality measure that can be applied across hospitals and providers. To the extent that "good" hospitals record complications more often than "bad" hospitals, such good hospitals look inferior when the complication rate is used as an outcome measure. As the adoption of the electronic medical record increases, especially in cardiovascular anesthesiology, such problems of recording should diminish. However, until the time when all anesthesiology suites have such equipment, differences in anesthesia recording will influence complication measures.

Finally, even if a quality measure satisfies all aspects of an ideal outcome measure, the cost of data collection will always be an important variable when judging its desirability. If the data for an outcome measure are too expensive to collect, then the data will not be available on a large scale, and it will be more difficult to make inferences about quality of care across hospitals and providers.

FAILURE TO RESCUE: A CONDITIONAL OUTCOME MEASURE

In an attempt to improve on the characteristics of the outcome measures of death and complications, we have proposed the "failure to rescue" rate as an outcome measure. To better understand this outcome measure, let us consider the following problem.

Suppose we observed two hospitals, Hospital A and Hospital B, both with exactly the same death rates. We could say that both deliver equal quality of care, but on closer inspection, Hospital A had a high complication rate but a low rate of death after complications, while Hospital B had a low rate of complication but a high rate of death following complications. Which hospital provides better quality of care? The answer rests in a better understanding of why patients die after complications and why patients develop complications. It is helpful to think of the death rate as a function of the complication rate and the rate of death after complications, which we call failure to rescue.

Equation 1 below displays the probability of death in terms of conditional probabilities.

$$p(d) = p(c) * p(d \mid c) + p(\text{not } c) * p(d \mid \text{not } c) \quad (1)$$

where p(d) represents the probability of death, p(d | c) is the conditional probability of death given a complication, p(not c) is the probability of no complication, and p(d | not c) is the conditional probability of death when no complication occurs. Because, for most surgical procedures, we may assume that if nothing goes wrong, the patient should not die, we can rewrite Equation 1 as:

$$p(d) = p(c) * p(d \mid c) \quad (2)$$

In other words, the death rate is defined as the complication rate multiplied by the failure to rescue rate (the failure rate).

The failure rate is a measure that focuses on how complications were handled by the hospital and provider. It de-emphasizes the cause of the complication, in part because complications are often difficult to predict, difficult to model, and are highly related to patient characteristics. Because the death rate is also a function of complications (see Equations 1 and 2), it becomes clear that the mortality rate is tainted with the same problems associated with complications. If, for example, complications were highly associated with patient factors, then mortality would also be associated with patient characteristics. To the extent that unobserved severity leads to complications, that same unobserved severity will lead to mortality; hence, the mortality measure will reflect a biased picture of hospital or provider quality.

There are many instances in which patient factors drive the complication rate more than hospital or provider factors. When observing common procedures that display much interhospital practice homogeneity before a complication, we may expect little influence of hospital or provider actions on the complication rate. In such circumstances, the variability in outcome is a function of how the complications were managed, not whether the patients developed complications.

One may believe that institutions that provide good quality of care will also have low death rates, low complication rates, and low failure rates. In other words, a good hospital should both prevent complications (relative to other hospitals) and prevent deaths (relative to other hospitals). Hence, failure to rescue would be an unnecessary quantity because, if there is good correlation between hospital death and complication rates, there must, by definition, be good correlation between hospital failure and complication rates and failure and death rates. However, as shown in Table 1–4, the correlation between hospitals ranked by their adjusted mortality and adjusted complication rates[15] is very poor. Most studies have shown correlations between hospital death and complication rates of <0.25. Obviously, the hospitals that prevent complications are not the same hospitals that prevent death, or at least the data suggest that. In a study on CABG surgery that we conducted,[7] there was poor correlation between death and complication rankings after adjusting for patient severity of illness. Figure 1–1 displays the rank correlation between death and complication rates in the 57 hospitals in that study. Some have argued that these poor correlations are due to differences in dimensions of quality across hospitals.[13]

TABLE 1–4. CORRELATION BETWEEN HOSPITAL RANKS: DEATH AND COMPLICATION

Study	Procedure/Condition	Hospitals (n)	r
Flood and Scott[8]	General surgical	17	−0.10
Silber et al.[15]	General surgical	142	0.21
Iezzoni et al.[10]	Major surgical	340	−0.01
Hartz et al.[19]	CABG	26	0.48
Hartz et al.[20]	CABG	10	0.31
Silber et al.[7]	CABG	57	0.07
DesHarnais et al.[21]	Medical and surgical	300	−0.05
Brailer et al.[13]	Medical and surgical	50	0.09

Data taken from Reference 15.
CABG, coronary artery bypass grafting.

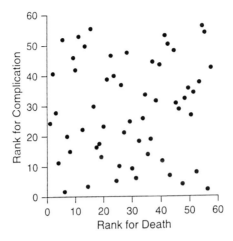

FIGURE 1–1. Correlation between the ranking of 57 hospitals using the adjusted death rate versus the adjusted complication rate. The Spearman correlation coefficient is 0.07 (P = 0.58). Data taken from Reference 7.

We believe that such poor correlation is due to either differences in either the failure rate (as a measure of quality of care) or unobserved severity (missing or omitted data).[15]

Much research has pointed to three aspects of the complication rate that would support avoiding its isolated use as a quality of care measure across hospitals. First, complications are highly driven by patient characteristics.[7,14,17,22] Table 1–5 provides the results of three logistic regression models predicting death, complication, and failure in elderly cholecystectomy and transurethral prostatectomy patients treated across seven states in 1985.[17] Each model is comprised of identical regression variables. The patterns of coefficients in these regressions display a common finding when comparing death, complication, and failure rates. Complications are highly related to patient characteristics, as observed by the larger odds ratios corresponding to patient variables. Second, we observe that failure is less a function of patient characteristics than are death or complication, except for history of cancer (presumably providers do not work as hard to salvage patients with cancer after complications as they would patients without cancer). Finally, we observe that failure is dependent on some hospital characteristics; in particular, on the board certification of the anesthesiology staff. The higher the percentage of board-certified anesthesiologists on staff, the lower the rate of death after complications.

In a second study comparing the outcomes of death, complication, and failure in an adult population of general surgical patients, complications and deaths were about 300 times more influenced by patient fac-

TABLE 1-5. THE RELATIVE RISKS (95% CONFIDENCE INTERVALS) FOR DEATH RATE, ADVERSE OCCURRENCE RATE, AND FAILURE RATE USING MULTIPLE LOGISTIC REGRESSION

	Outcome Measures		
	Death (n = 5972)	Adverse Occurrence (n = 5972)	Failure (n = 864)
Hospital characteristics			
High technology	0.51 (0.3, 0.9)[†]	0.94[b] (0.8, 1.1)	0.75 (0.4, 1.4)
Number of hospital beds	1.05 (0.8, 1.4)	1.07 (0.97, 1.2)	0.88 (0.6, 1.3)
Board-certified anesthesiologists (%)[a]	0.76 (0.6, 0.98)[*]	0.97 (0.9, 1.1)	0.63 (0.5, 0.9)[‡]
Board-certified surgeons (%)[a]	0.87 (0.22, 1.26)	0.86 (0.8, 0.99)[*]	1.37 (0.8, 2.2)
Presence of housestaff			
Surgical	1.44 (0.9, 2.4)	0.97 (0.8, 1.2)	2.05 (1.1, 3.9)[*]
Anesthesia	1.44 (0.8, 2.7)	1.05 (0.8, 1.3)	1.25 (0.6, 2.4)
Patient characteristics			
Age[a]	1.50 (1.2, 1.7)[∥]	1.21 (1.0, 1.3)[∥]	1.34 (1.1, 1.6)[§]
Male	1.04 (0.6, 1.4)	1.41 (1.2, 1.7)[∥]	0.82 (0.5, 1.5)
Cholecystectomy	2.01 (1.2, 3.5)[†]	2.83 (2.3, 3.4)[∥]	1.24 (0.6, 3.0)
History of Metastasis	3.95 (1.6, 10)[§]	1.08 (0.6, 2.0)	5.71 (1.6, 21)[‡]

Diabetes mellitus	1.29 (0.7, 2.7)	1.27 (1.02, 1.6)*	0.91 (0.5, 1.9)
Stroke	1.34 (0.7, 2.8)	1.69 (1.3, 2.3)‖	1.27 (0.6, 2.9)
Congestive heart failure	1.85 (1.0, 3.5)	1.78 (1.3, 2.4)‖	1.57 (0.7, 3.3)
COPD	1.63 (0.9, 3.0)	1.52 (1.2, 1.9)‖	0.90 (0.4, 2.0)
Admission severity score			
1	0.88 (0.5, 1.7)	1.45 (1.9, 2.9)‖	1.00 (0.5, 2.2)
2	1.77 (1.0, 3.3)	2.36 (1.9, 2.9)‖	0.89 (0.4, 1.9)
3 or 4	3.13 (1.5, 6.6)‖	4.25 (3.5, 5.8)‖	0.99 (0.4, 2.5)
Model χ^2 P value	0.0001	0.0001	0.0019
C-statistic	0.78	0.72	0.70

Data taken from Reference 17.
COPD = chronic obstructive pulmonary disease.
*$P < 0.05$.
†$P < 0.025$.
‡$P < 0.01$.
§$P < 0.005$.
‖$P < 0.001$.
^aThe relative risk is calculated for a 33% incremental change in the percentage of board-certified physicians and a 5-year incremental change in age.
^bNot significant—confidence intervals include 1.00.

tors than by hospital factors, whereas failure to rescue was about 90 times more influenced by patient factors than by hospital factors ($P = 0.05$ death versus failure).[23] This finding is illustrated in Figure 1–2, which displays three plots: one for death, one for complication (adverse occurrence), and one for failure. In each plot, the vertical distance from zero depicts the increased odds (positive) or decreased odds (negative) of dying (or developing a complication or failing) according to hospitals' characteristics along the base 2 log scale, so that 0 implies an odds ratio of 1, 1 implies an odds ratio of 2, 2 implies an odds ratio of 4, and 3 implies an odds ratio of 8. The horizontal axis depicts the patient components, with a positive number associated with patient characteristics that increase the chance of a bad outcome and a negative number associated with the odds of decreasing the chance of a bad outcome. An ideal outcome measure would be greatly influenced by hospital characteristics and would be only mildly influenced by patient characteristics; hence, the graph should be widely dispersed along the vertical axis and closely clustered along the horizontal axis. However, we observe the opposite pattern. There is great dispersion in outcomes with regard to patient characteristics, yet little dispersion across hospital characteristics. In other words, it appears that the variability in outcomes is far more influenced by patient characteristics than by hospital characteristics. It would seem that it is better to be well and to go to a poorly equipped hospital than to be sick and to go to the best equipped hospital, because the impact on outcome from hospital characteristics is far less than that from patient characteristics. As previously mentioned, when we compare the relative impact of patient and hospital characteristics on outcome, we find a difference among death, complication, and failure outcomes, with patient characteristics being approximately 300 times more influential to outcome than hospital characteristics for deaths and complication outcomes in general surgery, and only 90 times more influential for failure. Hence, concentrating on how complications were managed by studying the failure rate, rather than concentrating on the presence of a complication or the occurrence of a death, may provide better insight into quality because failure is relatively less influenced by patient characteristics.

Construct validity, another desirable property of the ideal outcome measure, has been lacking in many studies of the complication rate, but it is usually present in failure and mortality. In the study of 57 bypass programs reported in the MedisGroups National Comparative Database for 1991–1992, the authors found plausible relationships between hospital characteristics and outcome for death and failure, yet implausible relationships for complications.[7] For example, increased nurse to bed ratios, the presence of magnetic resonance imaging facilities, tertiary teaching center, and bone marrow transplantation units were all

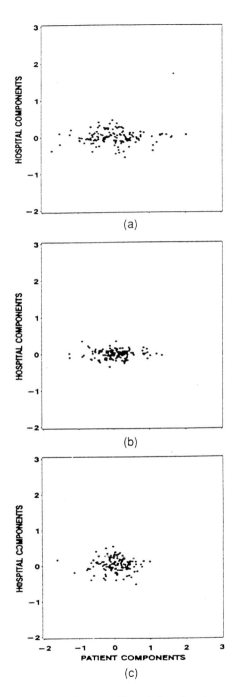

FIGURE 1–2. Relative contribution of hospital and patient components. *a*, death. *b*, adverse occurrence. *c*, failure. Data taken from Reference 23.

associated with higher complications rates but average or lower than average failure and death rates. Such findings should cause us to carefully choose our outcome measures and to avoid using measures (such as the complication rate) that appears to rank order hospitals in inverse relationship to hospital characteristics that indicate better quality of care.

Returning to the question asked at the beginning of this section: should we refer our patients to Hospital A or to Hospital B for their bypass surgery? A believer in failure to rescue would choose Hospital A. Such a hospital probably has a high complication rate because it has sicker patients with unobserved severity. As indicated by our studies, complications are highly patient-driven, and we would not fault Hospital A for its relatively high complication rate, yet we would salute it for maintaining its death rate at the same level as Hospital B, despite the more difficult patient population (as reflected by its increased complication rate).

Of course, such a use of the failure rate may be misleading if there were truly differences in hospital or provider abilities in avoiding complications after adequate severity adjustment. In such an instance, or if there were great differences in recording complications, it is useful to look at both the complication and the failure to rescue rates. Whenever complications may provide meaningful information on quality, it is be helpful to look at death, complication, and failure rates. If some hospitals intentionally underreport complications, the failure rate will be high in relation to a specified death rate. Gaming the system by underreporting or overreporting complications is much more difficult when all three measures are reported.

There are a number of potential benefits to using the failure to rescue measure. 1) Failure describes an aspect of care different from that described by the death rate or the complication rate, that being the ability of the hospital or provider to salvage patients after complications. This is beneficial when the complication rate—and, therefore, the death rate—is a function of patient characteristics, an undesirable attribute for a quality of care measure. 2) Failure may be less influenced by errors in severity adjustment, because all patients studied in the failure rate have experienced a complication. Therefore, failure has a built-in severity correction. 3) Failure may provide a check on complication rates that are underreported or inflated. Hospitals are less likely to game their data when all three rates are reported. Upcoding of patient severity may also be more difficult when all three rates are reported. Patients with high severity would generally be expected to have increased complications. A hospital can falsely underreport adjusted complication rates associated with lower than expected mortality (because of upcoding) and still have normal or increased failure rates because failure is less influenced by upcoding errors in severity adjustment, thereby lessening the upcoding problem.

UPCODING BIAS IN QUALITY STUDIES OF CARDIOVASCULAR SURGERY

Outcomes research studies on quality of care in cardiovascular surgery have lead the way for all quality studies in medicine.[24] In this section, I discuss some shortcomings in what are considered some of the best outcomes research initiatives in health services research. I briefly describe these studies and then critique them to convey some of the complexities encountered when conducting such research.

The best known outcomes research effort is probably the development of the Cardiac Surgery Reporting System (CSRS) by the New York State Department of Health.[25,26] Over the past decade, New York has lead the way in developing methodology to rank hospitals and providers. This effort generated the first published physician-specific mortality outcome reports. The New York State program is built around a predictive model of outcome based on physiologic variables recommended by an appointed State Cardiac Advisory Committee. Predictive variables include age, unstable hemodynamic state or shock, comorbidities (chronic obstructive pulmonary disease, diabetes, renal failure), ventricular function, and previous open heart operations. The observed mortality for hospitals and providers is then compared with the predicted mortality based on the model, and ranks (and ratings) are constructed accordingly. This methodology was criticized by Green and Wintfeld[27] because, among other problems, there appears to have been significant upcoding on the part of surgeons who reported the patient-specific prognostic factors. As shown in Table 1–6, the rates of reported congestive heart failure, renal dysfunction, and chronic obstructive pulmonary disease all increased at a rate well beyond plausible levels as the predictive models incorporated

TABLE 1–6. UPCODING SEVERITY

Risk Factor	Reported Prevalence (%)		
	1989	1990	1991
Renal failure	0.4	0.5	2.8
Congestive heart failure	1.7	2.9	7.6
Chronic obstructive pulmonary disease	6.9	12.4	17.4
Unstable angina	14.9	21.1	21.8
Low ejection fraction (<40%)	18.9	23.1	22.2

Data based on Reference 27.

these variables into the estimated mortality figures reported by the CSRS. In 1990, CSRS reports comparing death rates were distributed to the participating hospitals and published in the New York newspapers. As hospital risk-adjusted mortality rates were publicized, the reporting of patient risk factors also rose sharply. During this time period, the criteria for the definition of various risk factors also changed such that patients presenting with less severe symptoms were included in the increased risk groups. For example, the criterion for congestive heart failure was changed from "intractable" congestive heart failure to "signs" of congestive heart failure, and the criterion for renal failure was expanded from dependence on dialysis to a serum creatinine concentration >2.5 mg/dL.[27] Although this may have represented a change from underreporting in an era before cardiothoracic surgeons understood the importance of the New York State model, it is concerning that these rates were unstable. Whether upcoding significantly influences recent New York State reports remains to be proven. The upcoding may have been reduced in recent years; moreover, it may be uniform across hospitals and therefore may not influence across-hospital comparisons.

A similar problem, which may result in more significant bias, involves upcoding of the patient's severity of illness. This may be at play in a very well known study of quality improvement in CABG surgery in northern New England. O'Connor et al.[3,4], with the Northern New England (NNE) Cardiovascular Disease Study Group, reported a remarkable 24% decline in risk-adjusted mortality between 1987 and 1993 after instituting an extensive quality initiative in 1991–1992. The initiative, which included 23 cardiothoracic surgeons practicing in Maine, New Hampshire, and Vermont, collected data on 15,095 consecutive patients undergoing isolated CABG procedures during the study period and reported as its primary outcome measure a comparison of the observed and expected mortality rates. The initiative purportedly saved 74 lives over the study period.[4] This study was criticized by Ghali et al.[28] because it lacked a control group. Ghali et al.[28] showed that overall CABG mortality rates declined as much in Massachusetts as in NNE during the NNE study period, even though there was no quality initiative in Massachusetts. Ghali et al.'s critique has its own weaknesses, however: the Massachusetts data were based on the Massachusetts Health Data Consortium claims and did not include physiologically based variables, and it lacked the detail of the NNE study. However, there is another serious potential bias in the NNE study that has not been previously examined.

To understand the potential bias surrounding the results of the NNE study, it is important to understand its design. A prospective data collection effort was instituted by a collection of CABG programs throughout northern New England. It was observed that mortality following bypass varied considerably across institutions, and the authors decided that a cooperative effort to better understand this observation was in order. In 1991, O'Connor et al.[3] reported the risk adjustment model used in the NNE study. Variables in the risk-adjustment model included age, sex, body surface area, comorbidity score based on the Charlson Index, reoperation, low ejection fraction, left ventricular end-diastolic pressure, and emergent or urgent surgery (priority score). The priority score was assessed by the surgeon and was defined as follows:

> Emergent: medical factors relating to the patient's cardiac disease indicate that surgery should be performed within hours to prevent morbidity or death. This case should take precedence in time over an elective case, cause a new operating room to be opened, or be done at night or on a weekend if necessary. Urgent: medical factors require the patient to stay in the hospital to have the operation done before discharge. The risks of immediate morbidity and death are low. The patient would not necessarily take precedence over an elective case and could possibly wait for several days. Elective: medical factors indicate the need for operation, but the clinical picture allows discharge from the hospital with readmission at a later date.

It is of interest that in the initial model, the priority variable had the second largest impact on outcome, with only age contributing more to the chance of dying.[3]

The potential upcoding bias may be apparent when we observe the rate of urgent and emergent procedures versus elective procedures over the time of the study. The rate of urgent/emergent procedures increased from 53.6% to 59%. This was especially important because the authors stated that the benefit from the intervention occurred predominantly in the urgent/emergent priority group. In fact, without the urgent/emergent patients, there was no significant difference in mortality between the pre- and postintervention groups.

A potential bias arises from the use of a somewhat subjective priority score in the predictive model. As the Will Rogers joke goes, "When the Okies left Oklahoma and moved to California, the IQ of both states rose." By reclassifying (upcoding) elective patients to urgent/emergent status, the cardiac surgeons would improve both the statistics of the elective group (because the most difficult elective cases are now in the urgent/emergent group) and would also improve the urgent/emergent group (because the urgent/emergent group now includes less severe cases that previously were deemed elective). The influence of elective and urgent/emergent classification on outcomes are shown in Table 1–7.[4] There is great room to game the system by allowing surgeons to decide how to classify an important prognostic variable in the predictive model.

TABLE 1–7. OBSERVED AND EXPECTED DEATHS AND STANDARDIZED MORTALITY RATES DURING THE POSTINTERVENTION PERIOD

Patient Group	Observed Deaths (%)	Expected Deaths (%)	Observed-Expected Deaths	Standardized Mortality Ratio (95% Confidence Interval)	P^*
Male patients	145 (3.12)	179 (3.84)	−34	0.81 (0.68–0.94)	0.01
Female patients	89 (4.82)	129 (7.01)	−40	0.69 (0.55–0.83)	<0.001
Urgent/emergent	185 (4.83)	246 (6.41)	−61	0.75 (0.64–0.86)	<0.001
Elective	49 (1.84)	62 (2.33)	−13	0.79 (0.59–1.03)	0.11
Overall	234 (3.61)	308 (4.75)	−74	0.76 (0.67–0.90)	0.001

Data taken from Reference 4.
*Two-tailed P values are for observed versus expected deaths.

Let us assume that the Ghali et al.[28] analysis was correct and that the overall decline in NNE was due to general advances in CABG quality not specific to the NNE quality initiative. If we assume the nationwide improvement was exactly identical to the observed improvement in the NNE elective group, we can ask what the improvement in the urgent/emergent group would have been, assuming a Will Rogers effect. Based on the percentage of urgent/emergent versus elective patients in the prestudy group, approximately 350 of the 6488 patients in the study group were reclassified from elective to urgent/emergent. Of the 3010 potential elective cases, 350 may have been upcoded to urgent/emergent, leaving 2660 elective cases. To the 3478 urgent/emergent cases, we add the 350 previously elective cases, for a total of 3828 urgent/emergent cases. Starting with the assumed 19% reduction in mortality rate in patients undergoing elective surgery (from 2.33% to 1.89%), we can compute the associated reduction in urgent/emergent death rates as 6.41% prestudy to an estimated 5.19% poststudy. The NNE study reported a 4.83% mortality rate in the urgent/emergent group. If the 350 patients added to the urgent/emergent group had the same mortality rate as the remaining elective group, with a mortality rate of 1.89%, the addition of the 350 elective patients to the urgent/emergent group's mortality rate would have caused the urgent/emergent mortality to fall to 4.85%—a rate almost identical to the 4.83% mortality rate reported in the NNE study—solely because of the Will Rogers bias. Hence, secular trends as defined by Ghali et al.[28] and the Will Rogers bias can account for the improved mortality stemming from the NNE quality initiative.

It is important to point out that surgeons need not have consciously upcoded. In the New York State example, surgeons may simply have taken the prognostic variables more seriously. In the NNE case, surgeons concerned about improving outcome may have very reasonably shifted elective cases to urgent/emergent cases because they believed that this would improve mortality. From the perspective of policy makers and consumers assessing quality of care across hospitals and providers, however, these innocent and innocuous actions may have important effects on study results.

Although we cannot verify if any of the problems of bias noted in this section truly influenced any of the results of these studies, there is little doubt that the possibility of bias exists. One suggestion that could help to guard against such bias is to also report failure to rescue rates. Concentrating on those patients who developed complications may allow us to observe more stable outcome rates despite upcoding reclassification bias. As pointed out earlier, failure may be less susceptible to the bias noted in these studies because severity plays less of a role in determining death after complications than it does in the development of complications.

SUMMARY AND FUTURE RESEARCH

There is no doubt that good outcomes research provides information essential to a well functioning marketplace in all medical specialties, not excepting cardiovascular surgery. In this chapter, I attempted to define the necessary elements of the ideal outcome measure and, in so doing, to illustrate the challenges faced when using imperfect measures. The concept of failure to rescue was then introduced, and its strengths and limitations were discussed. With this in mind, potential upcoding bias was discussed, involving two very well known and influential initiatives in cardiovascular surgery. I suggested that reporting the failure rate may have aided in understanding whether the bias mentioned in this discussion was important. Clearly, more research is needed in our field to select better outcomes measures that are free of the potential limitations noted in this review. As the electronic medical and anesthesia record becomes more widely adopted, and as the variability in recording events diminishes, it will become easier to collect valid and uniform data across hospitals. This may lead to the development of better outcome measures. It will be the responsibility of the health services research community to ensure that these new outcome measures aid consumers and policy makers to make correct decisions so that market forces can optimize our healthcare, not erode it.

References

1. Hannan EL, Kilburn H, Racz M, Shields E, Chassin MR: Improving the outcomes of coronary artery bypass surgery in New York State. JAMA 271:761–766, 1994
2. Hannan EL, Siu AL, Kumar D, Kilburn H Jr, Chassin MR: The decline in coronary artery bypass graft surgery mortality in New York State: The role of surgeon volume. JAMA 273:209–213, 1995
3. O'Connor GT, Plume SK, Olmstead EM, Coffin CH, Morton JR, Maloney CT, Nowicki ER, Tryzelaar JF, Hernandez F, Adrian L, and the Northern New England Cardiovascular Disease Study Group: A regional prospective study of in-hospital mortality associated with coronary artery bypass grafting. JAMA 266:803–809, 1991
4. O'Connor GT, Plume SK, Olmstead EM, Morton JR, Maloney CT, Nugent WC, Hernandez F Jr, Clough R, Leavitt BJ, Coffin CH, Marrin CA, Wennberg D, Birkmeyer JP, Charlesworth DC, Malenka DJ, Quinton HB, Kasper JF: A regional intervention to improve the hospital mortality associated with coronary artery bypass graft surgery. JAMA 275:841–846, 1996

5. Silber JH, Rosenbaum PR: A spurious correlation between hospital mortality and complication rates: The importance of severity adjustment. Med Care 35:OS77–OS92, 1997
6. Messick S: Test validity and the ethics of assessment. Am Psychol 35:1012, 1980
7. Silber JH, Rosenbaum PR, Schwartz JS, Ross RN, Williams SV: Evaluation of the complication rate as a measure of quality of care in coronary artery bypass graft surgery. JAMA 274:317–323, 1995
8. Fleiss JL: Statistical methods for rates and proportions. 2nd ed. New York: John Wiley & Sons, 1981
9. Meier P: Terminating a trial: The ethical problem. Clin Pharmacol Ther 25:633–640, 1979
10. Iezzoni LI, Daley J, Heeren T, Foley SM, Hughes JS, Fisher ES, Duncan CC, Coffman GA: Using administrative data to screen hospitals for high complication rates. Inquiry 31:40–55, 1994
11. Iezzoni LI, Daley J, Heeren T, Foley SM, Fisher ES, Duncan C, Hughes JS, Coffman GA: Identifying complications of care using administrative data. Med Care 32:700–715, 1994
12. Iezzoni LI: Assessing quality using administrative data. Ann Intern Med 127:666–674, 1997
13. Brailer DJ, Kroch E, Pauly MV, Huang J: Comorbidity-adjusted complication risk: A new outcome quality measure. Med Care 34:490–505, 1996
14. Rosen AK, Geraci JM, Ash AS, McNiff KJ, Moskowitz MA: Postoperative adverse events of common surgical procedures in the Medicare population. Med Care 30:753–765, 1992
15. Silber JH, Rosenbaum PR, Williams SV, Ross RN, Schwartz JS: The relationship between choice of outcome measure and hospital rank in general surgical procedures: Implications for quality assessment. Int J Qual Health Care 9:193–200, 1997
16. Chassin MR, Park RE, Lohr KN, Keesey J, Brook RH: Differences among hospitals in Medicare patient mortality. Health Serv Res 24:1–31, 1989
17. Silber JH, Williams SV, Krakauer H, Schwartz JS: Hospital and patient characteristics associated with death after surgery: A study of adverse occurrence and failure to rescue. Med Care 30:615–629, 1992
18. Flood AF, Scott WR: Hospital structure and performance. Baltimore: Johns Hopkins University Press, 1987:174–206.
19. Hartz AJ, Kuhn EM, Green R, Rimm AA: The use of risk-adjusted complication rates to compare hospitals performing coronary artery bypass surgery or angioplasty. Int J Technol Assess Health Care 8:524–538, 1992
20. Hartz AJ, Kuhn EM, Kayser KL, Pryor DP, Green R, Rimm AA: As-

sessing providers of coronary revascularization: A method for peer review organizations. Am J Public Health 82:1631–1640, 1992
21. DesHarnais S, McMahon LF, Wroblewski R: Measuring outcomes of hospital care using multiple risk-adjusted indexes. Health Serv Res 26:425–445, 1991
22. Silber JH, Rosenbaum PR: Measuring quality of hospital care [letter]. JAMA 273:21–22, 1995
23. Silber JH, Rosenbaum PR, Ross RN: Comparing the contributions of groups of predictors: Which outcomes vary with hospital rather than patient characteristics? J Am Statis Assoc 90:7–18, 1995
24. Brook RH, McGlynn EA, Cleary PD: Measuring quality of care. N Engl J Med 335:966–970, 1996
25. Coronary artery bypass graft surgery in New York State 1990–1992. Albany: New York State Department of Health, December 1993.
26. Coronary artery bypass graft surgery in New York State 1989–1991. Albany: New York State Department of Health, December 1992.
27. Green J, Wintfeld N: Report cards on cardiac surgeons: Assessing New York State's approach. N Engl J Med 332:1229–1232, 1995
28. Ghali WA, Ash AS, Hall RE, Moskowitz MA: Statewide quality improvement initiatives and mortality after cardiac surgery. JAMA 277:379–382, 1997

Dennis M. Fisher

2 How Do We Obtain Outcome Data: Randomized Clinical Trials Versus Observational Databases

Areas of research in anesthesia have changed in recent years. Prior research efforts focused on topics such as the physiologic effects of anesthetic techniques or pharmacologic agents. These studies typically utilized small numbers of subjects, and statistical analysis was often descriptive or consisted of simple tests such as analysis of variance. As anesthetic and surgical techniques evolved such that perioperative risk is now minimal, and as society began to question the cost-benefit ratio of medical practice, the focus of medical research has shifted towards questions related to this cost-benefit ratio. Other medical specialties accepted these approaches a decade ago. For example, internists examined issues such as the cost-benefit ratio of a newer expensive antibiotic or the efficacy of single versus multiple doses of antibiotics. In recent years, the anesthesia community, led by pioneers such as Dennis Mangano, has asked similar questions about anesthesia care.

One problem inherent to outcomes research in anesthesia results from our great success in providing medical care without adverse outcomes. Consider a trial examining the efficacy of a new antibiotic to treat a resistant infection. If the traditional therapy failed in 40% of patients and we expected the new treatment to fail in <20% of patients (and its exorbitant cost could be justified only if its success rate attained this level or better), a power analysis reveals that a sample size of 128 patients (64 in each group) is sufficient to "assure" the success of a clin-

Outcome Measurements, edited by Kenneth Tuman. Lippincott Williams & Wilkins, Baltimore © 1999

ical trial (Table 2–1). One can readily expect the drug's manufacturer to sponsor two or more clinical trials with this number of patients.

In contrast, the anticipated outcome of anesthesia and surgery is success, and the expected failure rate—be it death, heart failure, or some other severe adverse outcome—is low. If the expected death rate after cardiac surgery were 1% and we wanted to show that an intervention improved this to 0.5% (probably an unrealistic increment in successful outcome when one considers the multifactorial nature of morbidity and mortality during anesthesia), a sample size of 7362 patients (3681 in each group) would be required. This leads to an obvious problem: who is willing to sponsor one or more trials of this magnitude?

In this chapter, I address five issues. First, I discuss the selection of outcomes; in particular, the implications of selecting a surrogate outcome. Second, I discuss my perspective on randomized clinical trials (RCTs) versus observational studies. Third, I comment on the use of meta-analysis as a tool to pool the results of potentially underpowered clinical trials. Fourth, I describe a conceptual approach to selection of sample size. Finally, I address some common statistical problems. The reader should recognize that my bias is toward RCTs and against meta-analysis.

This chapter is not designed as a comprehensive primer to guide researchers in research design. Rather, its purpose is to provide an introduction that both researchers and "users" can use to assist in developing clinical trials or critically assessing published or unpublished materials. I believe that the critical reader of the medical literature will be better equipped to judge the quality of medical research if issues regarding research design and analysis are more thoroughly understood.

SELECTING AN OUTCOME OR SURROGATE OUTCOME

A clinically based specialty such as anesthesia generates many interesting questions. For example, clinicians question whether a new anti-

TABLE 2–1. SAMPLE SIZES NEEDED TO DETECT A 50% DECREASE IN THE INCIDENCE OF AN ADVERSE EVENT WITH P VALUE OF 5% AND 80% POWER

Incidence in Control Group	Number per Group
40%	64
10%	342
1%	3681

emetic improves the patient's course of treatment relative to postoperative nausea and vomiting (PONV) or whether a drug administered during cardiopulmonary bypass improves the perioperative course of patients undergoing coronary artery bypass grafting. Although there are many important questions with regard to clinical anesthesia, I use these as examples of statistical analyses.

The incidence of PONV in control (typically, placebo) groups ranges from 20% to 70%, and treatment with various drugs may decrease this occurrence by 20%. In contrast, the incidence of perioperative myocardial infarction (MI) in control groups is much less, probably 1%–5%. This difference in the incidence of the adverse events in the control group has significant implications for study design. If the investigator expects that the treatment (i.e., the drug or monitoring device or any invention that distinguishes a group from the control group) improves outcome twofold, the expected frequency of vomiting of 50% in the control group may decrease to 25% with treatment; similarly, the incidence of MI may decrease from 1% in the control group to 0.5% with treatment. The sample size needed to demonstrate statistical significance differs between these two outcomes and may be prohibitive for the MI endpoint (Table 1–1) but not for the PONV endpoint. Rather than excluding the MI issue as untestable, the investigator may choose to study a surrogate outcome measure instead. For MI, a surrogate outcome might be the incidence of electrocardiographic (EKG) changes consistent with ischemia. In certain instances, a surrogate marker may be desirable not because it occurs more frequently, but because it can be measured more readily. For example, costs of medical care are often difficult to assess, but charges can be quantified more easily.

An ideal surrogate marker is one that is easy to measure and that is sufficiently frequent to permit the study to be conducted with a reasonable sample size. A second consideration is that changes in the incidence of surrogate measures must reflect changes in the incidence of the true measure. If, under a variety of circumstances, 20% of patients who showed EKG signs of ischemia developed MI, it may be wise to study the incidence of EKG changes rather than that of MI. However, if one anesthetic method led to frequent EKG changes but not to MI, whereas another technique led to the same frequent incidence of EKG signs and frequent MI, studies involving the surrogate outcome should not be extrapolated to predict the incidence of the true outcome.

It seems logical to assume that the percentage of patients free of PONV correlates well with patient satisfaction. Several factors mitigate against this correlation.[1] First, antiemetics may cause adverse effects that diminish their usefulness. A recent example is Tramèr et al.'s study,[2] which shows that although ondansetron decreases the incidence of PONV, it increases the incidence of headache and abnormalities in liver enzymes. Second, an analysis in which the occurrence of vomiting is treated dichotomously fails to distinguish between a patient with a single minor episode of vomiting 10 min after arrival in the postanesthesia care unit (to whom this episode is of little or no consequence) and another with persistent vomiting that delays discharge 2 h later. If the true motivation to decrease the incidence of PONV is to improve patient satisfaction or to decrease the incidence of prolonged in-hospital recovery (rather than, for example, to decrease the soiling of linen), then the adverse effects of treatment may be sufficient to overcome or even overwhelm any potential benefits. However, if the intent is to measure costs (including the soiling of linen or nursing activities related to cleaning patients), then all episodes of vomiting may need to be equally weighed.

A commonly used and problematic surrogate marker is hospital charges instead of costs. One such study examined whether (nonrandomized) extubation in the operating room versus the intensive care unit decreased hospital charges.[3] Because the hospital's policy was to charge separately for ventilatory support provided before and after midnight, a patient who arrived in the intensive care unit (ICU) 1 h before midnight and was extubated 1.5 h later would be charged for 2 days of support, whereas another patient ventilated for 12 h but extubated before midnight would be charged for only 1 day. Thus, despite the first patient using far fewer resources, the idiosyncrasies of the accounting system resulted in higher changes for that patient. In that hospitals charge in a manner quite inconsistent with costs (which insurance companies now recognize and reimburse hospitals for accordingly), it seems imprudent to perform any analysis using charges rather than costs.

Perhaps most problematic in the use of surrogate outcomes is the failure of investigators to identify them as such. Many studies of PONV claim that a decreased incidence of PONV should lead to a decreased incidence of unanticipated hospital admission, fewer prolonged recovery room stays, and improved patient satisfaction. Yet, many of these studies do not measure these outcomes, but instead count the incidence of patients free of PONV, despite a lack of studies that demonstrate the association of the surrogate and true outcomes.

Despite my criticism of the use of surrogate outcomes in anesthesia research,[1] there are instances in which their use is inevitable. The most obvious of these is when the incidence of the true outcome is so small in the treatment group that no reasonable sample size would attain statistical significance. However, whenever a surrogate outcome is used, the investigator should acknowledge its use and the resulting limitations. Although the expected more frequent occurrence of the surrogate outcome makes it more likely that the investigator will demonstrate statistical significance, the investigator must be cautious not to extrapolate a positive finding with the surrogate outcomes to one regarding the true outcome.

RANDOMIZED CLINICAL TRIALS

Historically, most clinical studies in anesthesia were RCTs. There were several advantages to this approach. First, the investigator could control the design precisely, thereby ensuring that the resulting data would allow for examination of the area in question. Second, the study could be both randomized and blinded, which are vitally important to minimize bias. Third, the investigator could perform a power analysis before conducting the study to determine the number of study subjects required to ensure sufficient power.

Randomization and Blinding

The hallmark of a RCT is that, if possible, both the investigator and the patient are blinded to the treatment to which each patient is assigned. In addition, treatments are assigned using some type of randomization procedure. These approaches minimize the opportunity for bias. Although investigators may claim that their nonrandomized, nonblinded studies are not biased, it is often difficult for them to demonstrate this convincingly. Bias can be introduced to studies in many subtle ways. In a well publicized violation of the design of a multicenter trial of therapy for breast cancer, one investigator abandoned certain enrollment criteria because of a personal belief that treatment was effective.[4,5] Had this violation not been identified by the study's coordinators, the results of the study may have been compromised. During the enrollment interview for an anesthesia study, a patient may report being at higher risk for a postoperative complication under investigation. If the investigator is aware of the group assignment, he/she may provide subtle clues that may influence the patient's willingness to participate.

Unless there are compelling reasons why a trial cannot be both randomized and blinded, both should be demanded from investigators in the formulation of study design.

Single-Center Versus Multicenter Trials

Occasionally, the investigator designing a study may determine that a RCT in his/her institution could not enroll sufficient subjects to demonstrate statistical significance, even if the study was conducted for years.

Demonstrating an improvement in adverse outcomes from 1.0% to 0.5% requires >7000 patients, certainly a daunting task. In response, the investigator may invite 9 or 99 other investigators to participate, thus decreasing the number of subjects per center from 7362 to 736 or 74. The latter number is certainly closer to the range of sample sizes that one could obtain in a reasonable time frame, making the multicenter approach desirable. The multicenter approach assures a greater likelihood that the study will be conducted more rapidly, but it also incurs risks. Perhaps most significant of these risks (because of its subtlety) is the possibility that individual centers will deviate from the protocol in ways that influence outcome but are not identified by the investigators.

Once the decision is made to involve more than a single center in a trial, several problems appear. An obvious issue is that the results may differ among institutions, a result of differences in patient population, surgical technique, surgical skills, or other covariates. For example, a new therapy (which we "know" to be effective) may be designed to decrease perioperative blood loss in patients undergoing cardiac surgery. Figure 2–1 displays simulated data from three centers in which this therapy was compared with a placebo group. Within each center, the effect of the treatment is apparent, and statistical significance is attained, despite a small sample size. However, a pooled analysis (as would be the statistical approach used to analyze this multicenter trial) fails to demonstrate statistical significance, a result of large between-center dif-

Outcome Studies: RCT's *vs*. Observational Databases

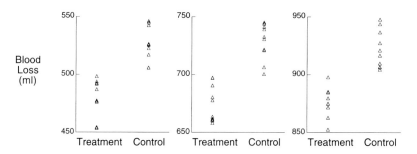

FIGURE 2–1. Simulated data from a three-center clinical trial. Each panel displays measured blood loss in two groups of 10 patients. The control group at each center received a placebo, and the treatment group received a therapeutic agent designed to decrease blood loss. When data for the three centers are pooled, statistical significance is not attained. However, within each center, the data demonstrate statistical significance. This example illustrates how increasing sample size by increasing the number of sites included in a study may not necessarily improve (and, as in this simulated instance, may actually worsen) statistical power.

ferences in blood loss in both the control and treatment groups. Thus, although the multicenter approach offered rapid collection of data, it compromised the results. Fortunately, statistical techniques (in this instance, a linear data transform) exist to rectify this particular problem. The average value for blood loss at each center can be subtracted from the value for each subject. This approach, termed "centering the data," would improve the statistical power of the analysis. However, statistical manipulations of this sort should be adopted *a priori*, i.e., before initiation of the study.

Tight Versus Loose Control of Studies

The implications of tight versus loose control of experimental conditions should be considered. For example, one may conduct a study in which vigorous attempts were made to control blood pressure in both the treatment and control groups versus one in which a significantly wider (yet still clinically acceptable) range of blood pressures was allowed in both groups. The incidence of adverse outcomes (the focus of this study) may be markedly lower in both the treatment and control groups in which blood pressure was well controlled. Although this may lead to the conclusion that tight control of blood pressure is desirable to minimize adverse outcomes, that was not the stated goal of this study. However, adverse events may be so infrequent in the groups with tight control that one may not be able to demonstrate a benefit to the treatment under investigation. If tight control is realistic only in a research setting, then application of the results of this trial to the clinical environment may be limited.

Large Databases

In many situations, the ability to conduct a RCT is limited. For example, the projected sample size may be so large as to make the cost of a study prohibitive. The potential investigator may be unable to conduct a clinical trial but may have skills in data analysis. In these instances, another source of data for analysis may be observational databases. With the advent of electronic data collection, institutions such as hospitals, health care systems, regulatory bodies, and governmental agencies compile massive databases regarding healthcare outcomes that may be relevant to clinical research. For example, hospital or blood bank information systems may track all the blood that is administered to all patients. Governmental agencies may track all deaths that occur in each hospital and the reported cause of death. Frequently, these databases are available for research purposes.

The magnitude of these databases is seen by some investigators as providing unparalleled opportunities for research. Advocates of this approach note that the quantity of data available through existing databases probably cannot be matched, even at astronomic cost. In addition, these databases include information on actual clinical practice, rather than on the potentially altered practice used in research protocols (e.g., tight control).

Critics, however, cite numerous dilemmas. Foremost of these is that the information in these databases is not obtained in a prospective, randomized manner. One example of such research is a study that examines the differences among medical centers in the likelihood of death after cardiac surgery.[6] Those hospitals with poor outcomes argue that their complications resulted from caring for higher-risk patients. Investigators who perform these analyses frequently attempt to control for risk (for example, results can be stratified by age, accounting for possible differences in outcome for patients of different ages). Although these risk adjustments are claimed to be sufficient, it is doubtful whether they are. In contrast, the RCT design hopefully protects the investigator from introducing this problem.

Another example of the influence of lack of randomization can be seen in the comparison of two surgical approaches to the repair of coronary artery disease. In this fictitious example, investigators are unaware that the clinicians were interested in this same issue and that all high-risk patients underwent Procedure A, whereas lower-risk patients underwent Procedure B. The investigator obtained data from a hospital database, and the outcome measure is incidence of MI in the year after surgery. Although Procedure A is better (by definition), outcome is no different in the two groups because of differences in selection.

A second problem involves blinding, although I use the term differently than when referring to the RCT. It may be that the team caring for the patients is more interested in the outcome of patients undergoing Procedure A than in those undergoing Procedure B. therefore, all patients undergoing Procedure A are strongly encouraged to return for follow-up care (possibly even provided *gratis*). In turn, the percent follow-up in the two groups differs markedly. This undoubtedly influences the results. Although issues of surveys are quite different, the analogy to return rates for surveys is important—investigators are often satisfied that 50% of the individuals sent questionnaires returned them, yet are unable to comment on what distinguishes the 50% who did from those who did not!

A third problem involves an unidentified influence of time. In some cases, investigators examine the incidence of an outcome before and after the introduction of a new clinical practice. For example, a trial mentioned earlier[3] examined whether a new policy of extubating children in the operating room after cardiac surgery saved money compared with extubation in the ICU. The authors assume that the only factor that affected charges during the time period was the new extubation practice. The validity of this assumption is certainly questionable, even based on the data presented by these authors. In addition to the two groups already described (those patients studied before the change in practice who were not extubated in the operating room and those patients studied after the change in practice who were extubated in the operating room), the authors obtained data on a third group, patients studied after the change in practice who were not extubated in the operating room. Hospital charges for this group were markedly lower than those for the group studied in the earlier time period. Thus, the decreased charges in the early extubation group could be, at least partially, attributed to practice changes that occurred over time independent of the change in extubation practice.

A recent noncardiac study illustrates a similar situation. Macario et al.[7] found that the institution of practice guidelines decreased the costs of knee replacement by 19%. However, costs for a second procedure, prostatectomy, decreased 12% during the same time interval, despite no practice guidelines being instituted. Thus, only a portion of the savings can be attributed to the guidelines, a finding that could be identified only because the investigators selected an appropriate control group. Lack of such a control group markedly diminishes the validity of other similar studies. For example, Lubarsky et al.[8] reported that a pharmaceutical practice guideline in their institution decreased the cost of drugs used during anesthesia by $24. The authors dismissed a 7-min increase in anesthesia time as being of no consequence. This increase in anesthesia time may have resulted from changes in surgical practice, such as a greater number of laparoscopies and a decrease in open procedures, and may not have been a detrimental outcome from their pharmaceutical practice guidelines. However, the results of Macario et al.'s practice guideline study[7] and recent changes in practice in other university hospitals (e.g., the increased likelihood that an attending surgeon, rather than an undersupervised medical student, will perform skin closure) suggest that anesthesia time should have decreased rather than increased during the period of the study. Thus, the 7-min increase in anesthesia time may represent the tip of the iceberg. Lack of a control group prevents the investigators and their critics from determining the answer.

A fourth problem with the use of retrospective databases concerns the management of missing data. When data are collected prospectively, investigators can define *a priori* how missing data will be handled in the subsequent analysis. In addition, investigators can endeavor to minimize the quantity of data that is missing. In contrast, databases often lack large amounts of critical information. Excluding these missing data from a retrospective analysis may lead to a bias. For example, if investigators were examining survival with different anesthetic techniques, data missing at a 3-month follow-up visit may reflect either patients lost to follow-up (e.g., having moved to a new community or healthcare plan) or having died.

A fifth issue regards the quality of data. When investigators obtain data prospectively, they generally define criteria explicitly. For example, a study examining the influence of anesthetic technique on time to recovery room discharge may use strict criteria to define the time at which a patient is ready for discharge. In contrast, an existing database, such as a recovery room log, would provide data as to when the patient was actually discharged, rather than when the patient attained the criteria for discharge. Thus, potentially unrelated factors such as the availability of transportation may confound the results. In addition, the accuracy of the values entered for routine clinical tracking is often questionable.

Finally, the question of interest is probably not answered exactly by the database. For example, it is likely that the investigator has narrow questions of interest, yet those who created and implemented the database did not ask these specific questions. Under this scenario, investigators may choose to use other measures, such as surrogate outcomes. The compromise may be small, or it may be large.

Despite the marked cost-savings associated with retrospective studies involving databases, few, if any, of these studies have been accepted into the anesthesia literature, presumably a result of these serious limitations.

META-ANALYSIS: A SOLUTION OR A PROBLEM?

Frequently, as a clinical issue emerges, small clinical trials are conducted independently at a number of institutions. For example, numerous trials have studied the influence of antiemetics on the incidence of PONV. Some of these studies achieve statistical significance, whereas others suggest a trend, but a small sample size fails to demonstrate statistical significance. With the latter, investigators may conclude that the therapy was not beneficial. One prominent example in the anesthesia literature regards the influence of regional versus general anesthesia on outcomes in high-risk patients, an issue that has been examined in many small studies. The conflicting results of these multiple publications frustrates the clinician who tries to apply the results of these analyses. Although the optimal solution may be to perform a large RCT that is sufficiently powered to demonstrate statistical significance, several factors mitigate against the likelihood of this happening. First, the expense of such a trial may be prohibitive. Second, investigators may be concerned that efforts expended in the earlier trials will have been wasted. Finally, funding agencies may feel that the earlier trials provided sufficient evidence that the new trial is not warranted.

Under these circumstances, one currently popular approach is termed meta-analysis. With this technique, the investigator (henceforth identified as the meta-analyst) does not obtain data himself/herself. Rather, the meta-analyst carefully searches bibliographic databases to obtain a comprehensive list of relevant publications. Each study is then examined to determine its quality and suitability for inclusion in a pooled analysis. For example, studies in which the randomization procedure was not stated explicitly may be rejected. Statistical techniques specifically created for meta-analysis are then applied to the results of these studies, accounting for the different sample size in each study, to yield a pooled result—for example, an odds ratio. For example, a meta-analysis of the effects of regional versus general anesthesia for surgical repair of femoral neck fracture reported that general anesthesia was associated with a fourfold higher incidence of deep-vein thrombosis.[9]

Meta-analysis has polarized the medical research community. Its advocates claim that it is a legitimate method to resolve questions for which multiple inadequately powered studies have been performed, and its efficiency is appealing (in that existing studies are used, no additional patients are subjected to the less desirable therapy). In contrast, its critics claim that it is flawed. First, meta-analysts typically do not have access to the original data; therefore, the published data become their new database. Unfortunately, editorial constraints often prevent publication of vast amounts of data; therefore, the information available to the meta-analyst may be insufficient. In addition, issues that were well established and handled appropriately by the investigator may not be well defined in the manuscript, which prevents the meta-analyst from using the information correctly. The meta-analyst typically deals with these issues by assigning a quality score to each study and using only those studies that meet certain criteria. However, the procedure by which studies are judged as acceptable or unacceptable for inclusion is questionable—well designed studies may be rejected simply because the authors failed to specify certain criteria demanded by the meta-analyst (and such criteria may have been standard practice at the time that the study was conducted but not routinely reported).

Second, the database from which the trials are identified may be incomplete and, possibly, biased. This publication bias (or "file drawer" problem) occurs because an underpowered study that fails to demonstrate statistical significance is likely not to be published, whereas a similarly sized study that attains statistical significance is. Assuming that the former set of studies is inaccessible to the meta-analyst (and there are virtually no registries that collect these data), the meta-analysis will be biased toward studies with positive results. This problem is typically discounted by meta-analysts as unimportant, despite their inability to assess its prevalence. Finally, meta-analysis may include studies with different designs.

The test of meta-analysis, ultimately, is whether it yields the same results as an adequately powered, large RCT. Recently, LeLorier et al.[10] examined 40 primary and secondary outcomes for which such a comparison could be performed. In many instances, the large RCT yielded conclusions different from those of the meta-analysis, despite effect-size estimates that differed minimally (i.e., the magnitude of effect detected by the meta-analysis was similar to that detected by the large RCT, yet the meta-analysis yielded a different conclusion than the RCT). In this case, one may question whether the meta-analysis or the large RCT yielded the more meaningful result. Of course, the design of each of the many small RCTs and the large RCT must be compared. If there is no obvious difference between them, my bias would be toward the large RCT. In this context, many researchers are critical of meta-analysis.

DETERMINING THE NECESSARY SAMPLE SIZE

In some instances, an investigator will report a P value equal to 0.05 for a critical analysis. The implications of this P value should be considered. If one subject included in a study were replaced by another, it is likely that the results from these two subjects would differ. In turn, differences between the two groups would be either smaller or larger. If the difference were smaller, the P value would now be >0.05, and statistical significance would not be attained. In turn, the results of the study would diminish in importance.

To avert such problems, it is advisable for investigators to perform a power analysis before the study is initiated. This analysis permits the investigators to determine how many patients should be included to assure the study's success. Unfortunately, many studies are performed without an appropriate power analysis, and investigators frequently submit manuscripts in which small sample sizes yielded P values of 0.05–0.1 (5%–10%). In some instances, the investigators claim that these results indicate a trend (i.e., they imply statistical significance); in others, they claim that this P value indicates no difference between groups. In either instance, the inadequate sample size prevents the reviewer or reader from arriving at a meaningful conclusion. In response, it has become fashionable for reviewers to request a *post hoc* power analysis, i.e., to use the existing data to estimate how many patients should have been studied to attain statistical significance. If the P value were close to 0.05, then the results of this *post hoc* power analysis are obvious—the number of patients studied was inadequate, and a small increase in sample size (assuming that the data from the new subjects followed a pattern identical to that in the patients already studied) would be sufficient to attain statistical significance. If the P value was much larger than 0.05, then a considerably larger sample size would have been needed. This *post hoc* power analysis does not, however, provide any insights into the validity of the results or clinical implications of the present study. Thus, I remain skeptical of *post hoc* power analysis. Instead, power analyses should be performed before commencing the study.

In designing a study, one presumably has some idea of the result. For example, the incidence of EKG changes consistent with ischemia may be 30% with a common anesthetic agent, and one may expect an incidence of only 12% with a new agent (therefore, an effect size of 18%). The number of eligible patients may be 100 per year, and the investigator may be constrained to performing the study within 1 year (e.g., during a fellowship). A statistical analysis (either a continuity corrected χ^2 test or Fisher's exact test) based on these expected results yields a P value <0.05 (0.049 or 0.048, respectively). Therefore, the investigator may commence the experiment, confident that the results will turn out as expected and that statistical significance will be attained by the end of the experiment.

Luck may be with the investigator. After studying 100 patients, the incidence of adverse events may be exactly as planned, and statistical significance will have been attained. Or the situation may be even better—the incidence of ischemia may be only 10% in the treatment group and 30% in the control group (this results from only one fewer patient having ischemia in the treatment group), leading to a P value of 0.02. However, it is equally likely that the results could be unfavorable to the investigator's hypothesis. For example, the incidence of ischemia may be 14% in the treatment group and 30% in the control group (this results from a change in outcome for only a single patient!). Despite the effect size (16%) still being quite large, statistical significance is not attained ($P = 0.09$), and the investigator may conclude that the therapy is not effective (and may not even attempt to publicize the results). Another possibility is that the surgical team may vacation during the 12th month of the study, decreasing the sample size to 46 per group, and a P value of 0.08. Thus, with an experiment designed to achieve a P value of 0.05, trivial changes in the samples size and/or results lead either to success or failure with nearly equal frequency.

This leads to the concept of the power of the trial. The study described above and any study in which the expected results yield a P value of 0.05 exactly have a power of 50% (meaning that 50% of the time, the expected variability will lead to success and 50% of the time, to failure). Bettors may consider 50% to be good odds, but most researchers would not concur. Therefore, before investing any resources (time, money, pride), an investigator should decide how much power the trial has to answer the study question. Typically, an investigator selects a sample size sufficient to assure statistical significance with 80% power.

STATISTICAL ISSUES

There are several final considerations regarding statistical analysis of clinical trials. Statistical methods never determine "truth," but rather point us to those observations that are not likely to have occurred by chance. Because we accept a 5% chance that our statistically significant observation occurred by chance (i.e., may be by chance) when we use a P value of 0.05, we need to prepare our statistical analyses carefully. The most common error is to perform multiple statistical comparisons on the same data. If one accepts a 5% chance of being wrong with a single comparison, the chance of being wrong increases to nearly 10% with two comparisons and to 14% with three. Certainly, no one would be satisfied with claiming statistical significance if it were achieved at the 14% level! Yet, this occurs commonly.

A second problem with statistical analysis results from collecting too much data. If the investigator fails to achieve statistical significance of the primary question, it is tempting to select a whole series of new questions, performing unintended statistical analyses, an approach known as data torturing.[11] The legitimacy of this approach is certainly questionable.

SUMMARY

The decision to perform a RCT versus an analysis based on an observational database is often influenced by issues of financial and staff resources. Regardless of the decision made by the investigator, the disadvantages of the selected approach must be considered.

References

1. Fisher DM: Surrogate end points: Are they meaningful? Anesthesiology 81:795–796, 1994
2. Tramèr MR, Reynolds DJ, Moore RA, McQuay HJ: Efficacy, dose-response, and safety of ondansetron in prevention of postoperative nausea and vomiting: A quantitative systematic review of ran-

domized placebo-controlled trials. Anesthesiology 87:1277–1289, 1997
3. Laussen PC, Reid RW, Stene RA, Pare DS, Hickey PR, Jonas RA, Freed MD: Tracheal extubation of children in the operating room after atrial septal defect repair as part of a clinical practice guideline. Anesth Analg 82:988–993, 1996
4. Fisher B, Redmond CK: Fraud in breast-cancer trials [letter]. N Engl J Med 330:1458–1460, 1996
5. Poisson R: Fraud in breast-cancer trials [letter]. N Engl J Med 330:1460, 1994
6. Schneider EC, Epstein AM: Influence of cardiac-surgery performance reports on referral practices and access to care: A survey of cardiovascular specialists. N Engl J Med 335:251–256, 1996
7. Macario A, Horne M, Goodman S, Vitez T, Dexter F, Heinen R, Brown B: The effect of a perioperative clinical pathway for knee replacement surgery on hospital costs. Anesth Analg 86:978–984, 1998
8. Lubarsky DA, Glass PS, Ginsberg B, Dear GL, Dentz ME, Gan TJ, Sanderson IC, Mythen MG, Dufore S, Pressley CC, Gilbert WC, White WD, Alexander ML, Coleman RL, Rogers M, Reves JG: The successful implementation of pharmaceutical practice guidelines: Analysis of associated outcomes and cost savings. Anesthesiology 86:1145–1160, 1997
9. Sorenson RM, Pace NL: Anesthetic techniques during surgical repair of femoral neck fractures: A meta-analysis. Anesthesiology 77:1095–1104, 1992
10. LeLorier J, Gregoire G, Benhaddad A, Lapierre J, Derderian F: Discrepancies between meta-analyses and subsequent large randomized, controlled trials. N Engl J Med 337:536–542, 1997
11. Mills JL: Data torturing. N Engl J Med 329:1196–1199, 1993

Fredrick K. Orkin

3 | Application of Outcomes Research to Clinical Decision Making in Cardiovascular Medicine

Outcomes research is a new, rapidly evolving, multidisciplinary field that promises valuable guidance to anesthesiologists in their clinical decision making relating to cardiovascular medicine. In this chapter, I survey the new field, emphasizing what it is and how it may be applied. Since we can only sample the more salient aspects of outcomes research in a short chapter, many reference works have been included among the references.

At the outset, many anesthesiologists may ask what is so new about outcomes research, for *outcome* is so commonly used in our recent publications that it has become hackneyed. Yet, almost all usage of the term in our literature relates to *clinical outcomes.* For example, a recent review of anesthetic outcomes[1] adopted a revisionist perspective to provide seemingly comprehensive coverage but barely ventured beyond clinical outcomes. Similarly, an international workshop convened to improve outcome studies[2] provided a similarly limited view. *Outcomes research* refers to the study of a far broader array of phenomena related to care, of which clinical outcomes constitute but one subset. Indeed, so little outcomes research has been performed in relation to anesthesia that the prospects for enhanced decision making and substantial improvement of care are great. However, to appreciate what outcomes research offers, we must first understand how and why the field developed.

Outcome Measurements, edited by Kenneth Tuman. Lippincott Williams & Wilkins, Baltimore © 1999

THE EMERGENCE OF OUTCOMES RESEARCH

It has become trite to recount the almost unbridled growth in United States healthcare expenditures during the past 30 years. Yet, the emergence of outcomes research reflects a response to the growth of our healthcare sector at 2–3 times the growth in the general economy during most of this period, despite governmental and private sector initiatives to moderate the growth. At the same time, 15% of the population has been uninsured and thus has had limited access to healthcare, and population health indices (e.g., life expectancy, infant mortality) have lagged behind those of countries with lower per capita healthcare spending. This *feast and famine* circumstance increasingly has suggested misallocation of resources and a need to reform the healthcare system.[3] Viewed from the perspective of purchasers of care in the United States healthcare marketplace, there has been a growing need to achieve greater *value*,[4] which may be represented as

$$\text{Value} = \frac{\text{Quality}}{\text{Cost}}$$

That is, although the quality of care generally has seemed very good, the purchasers have felt that the care costs too much. Alternatively, the care should be even better for what is spent. However, healthcare providers have typically viewed quality and cost as closely linked, such that high-quality care requires very large expenditures and that controlling or lowering healthcare expenditures necessarily results in poorer quality of care.

Appropriateness of Care Analysis

Quality of care and healthcare cost are actually not closely linked, as demonstrated by two major bodies of research, both of which document the substantial variation in what physicians do under similar clinical circumstances. Underlying high-quality care is sound clinical judgment, by which is meant determining which interventions (or watchful waiting) lead consistently to net benefits for individual patients.[5]

One body of research, using the RAND-University of California at Los Angeles Delphi panel method,[6] has explored clinical judgment by evaluating the appropriateness of care. A panel of experts relating to a given disorder develop a set of explicit indications for a given procedure related to the disorder, and a large number of medical records of patients who had the specified procedure are audited for the presence of indications for the procedure. When the methodology is applied to patients undergoing cardiovascular procedures, such as carotid endarterectomy or coronary artery bypass graft (CABG) surgery, typically

14%–20% of the surgery has been deemed "inappropriate," depending on disease severity and other factors (Fig. 3–1).[7,8]

Such results have been considered a general measure of the overuse of medical technology, which, according to a congressional Office of Technology Assessment (OTA) definition, includes drugs, medical and surgical procedures, protocols, support systems, and organizational systems through which healthcare is delivered.[9] By extension, if inappropriate care can be wrung out of the healthcare system, patient outcomes (and quality) should be no worse, and substantial savings should be achieved. Very recently, however, variation has been demonstrated among the expert panels developing the indications, as well as between the panels and practicing physicians,[10,11] which highlights the "complex interplay of evidence, contexts or circumstances, and values or preferences"[5] that enter into clinical judgment. Yet, such variation in underlying indications is itself indicative of uncertainty about and lack of conclusive evidence for most clinical practices, which suggests (albeit in a roundabout way) that quality can be maintained while superfluous care and costs are decreased.

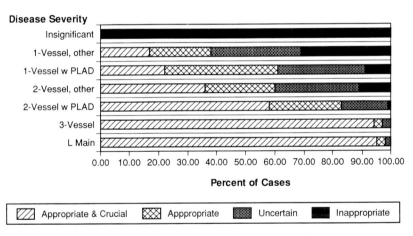

FIGURE 3–1. Appropriateness of coronary artery bypass graft surgery, by disease severity, in 1338 patients in New York State in 1990, using the RAND methodology. Disease severity was assessed by angiography, with a minimum of 50% narrowing in affected vessels, with the exception of cases in which "insignificant" narrowing was noted. PLAD, proximal left anterior descending artery. Whereas all procedures related to insignificant narrowing were deemed inappropriate, almost all procedures with moderate or severe pathology were judged appropriate. With <3% of CABG procedures performed for inappropriate reasons and 7% for uncertain reasons, these New York State results are considerably better than those reported in other sites (typically 14% and 30%, respectively) and have been attributed to the state's regulatory environment, which limits the number of sites at which the procedure is performed. Data taken from Reference 8.

Small-Area Variation Analysis

The second body of evidence suggesting that quality of care and healthcare cost are not closely linked involves a geographic approach. A large literature documents the substantial variation in use of healthcare technology and resources across small geographic areas, even closely neighboring communities with similar need for and access to services.[12,13] For example, the rate of CABG surgery in New Haven, CT was found to be twice that in Boston, MA, whereas the rate of carotid endarterectomy in Boston was about twice that in New Haven; however, the incidence of coronary artery disease was no greater, nor was the incidence of cerebrovascular disease any lower, in New Haven than in Boston.[14] Across the United States, there is an almost fourfold variation in the per capita rate of CABG surgery and more than sevenfold variation in the rate of carotid endarterectomy that is unexplained by the underlying rates of coronary and cerebrovascular disease (Fig. 3–2 and 3–3).[15] Such varia-

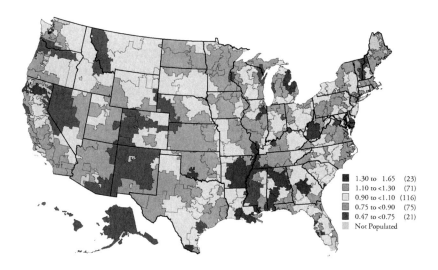

FIGURE 3–2. The variation in per capita rates of coronary artery bypass graft (CABG) surgery by hospital referral regions (HRR) across the United States compared with the national average rate, based on 1994–1995 Medicare data. Of the 306 regions, 23 had rates ≥30% higher than the national average, including parts of Alabama, Arkansas, California, Florida, and Michigan. Twenty-one regions had rates >25% below the national average; these included parts of the Northeast, mountain states, California, Alaska, and Hawaii. By HRR, the rate of hospitalization for acute myocardial infarction, a marker for coronary artery disease, and the rate of CABG surgery were uncorrelated ($R^2 = 0.005$). Reproduced with permission from Reference 15, page 115. © The Trustees of Dartmouth College.

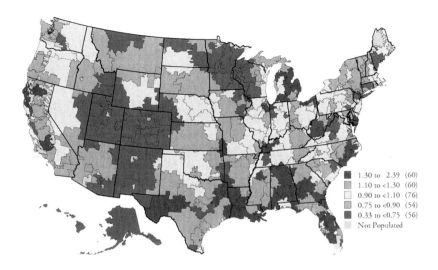

FIGURE 3–3. The variation in per capita rates of carotid endarterectomy by hospital referral regions (HRR) across the United States compared with the national average rate, based on 1994–1995 Medicare data. Of the 306 regions, 60 had rates ≥30% higher than the national average, including parts of California, Michigan, the deep South, and Florida. Fifty-six regions had rates >25% below the national average, including parts of New England, the plains and mountain states, and the Northwest. By HRR, the rate of hospitalization for stroke, a marker for cerebrovascular disease, and the rate of carotid endarterectomy were poorly correlated ($R^2 = 0.22$). Reproduced with permission from Reference 15, page 125. © The Trustees of Dartmouth College.

tion in surgical rates mirrors similar variation in the use of other healthcare resources, including numbers and types of healthcare personnel, hospital beds and other physical resources, and healthcare expenditures.[15]

These large variations in utilization of healthcare resources await explanation, despite substantial research that yielded no reasons (e.g., a high rate of CABG surgery associated with a high prevalence of thoracic surgeons). The variation is believed to reflect the effects of several factors: absence of documentation for the efficacy of perhaps 80% of medical technology, professional uncertainty about the indications for and value of specific technology (as noted above), availability of facilities and other resources with which to furnish the services (e.g., the availability of surgeons and operating rooms), and some degree of what economists call supplier-induced demand (i.e., healthcare providers are taught to provide a service rather than to deliberate and wait).[13]

As with inappropriate care identified by the RAND methodology, small-area variations are more than sociologic phenomena. Such variation exists without apparent health benefit in high-use areas or related health problems in low-use areas.[15] Moreover, the arguably superfluous care—whether performed in a high-use area or deemed inappropriate—engenders additional societal costs, including direct expenditures for care, indirect costs (e.g., time lost from work), and the medical and social sequelae associated with surgical and anesthetic-related complications. Given the inherent rate of complications among procedures, the decision to perform surgery in individual cases in high-use areas may be a more important determinant of patient outcome than how well the procedure is performed.[16]

The Economist's Production Function

Further insights into the relationship between quality of care (or patient outcome or benefit) and healthcare expenditures may be gleaned from the economist's production function, which describes a relationship between overall health benefit and incremental inputs to healthcare (Fig. 3–4A).[17,18] As in other productive endeavors, the anesthesiologist should continue to add resources (e.g., newer, more costly drugs; special patient monitoring devices; pain management protocols) to care as long as there is additional benefit. Beyond the top of the curve, the point of maximal benefit and, thus, optimal investment, further investment merely results in *negative* benefit (e.g., complications, higher cost without patient benefit). Whereas it is commonly believed that the American healthcare system has passed the top of the curve, we may rationalize our situation by selectively reducing investment where appropriate and moving back to the point of maximal benefit (Fig. 4B).

Although the economist's production function may seem arcane, this construct applies well to many decisions that anesthesiologists face. These decisions run the gamut from drug choice and equipment acquisition to administrative policies relating to organizing and delivering care. In each, the challenge is choosing appropriate technology (recognizing the broad Office of Technology Assessment definition[9]) and using technology appropriately.

Cost-Effectiveness Analysis

The challenge of knowing that we are doing what is appropriate (no more, no less) is especially difficult. The principal problem is that our knowledge of the effectiveness of our technology, among other complex

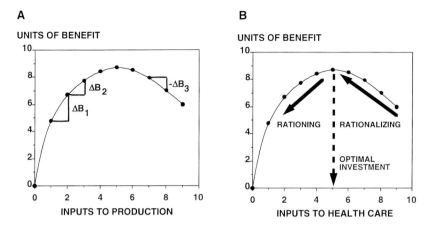

FIGURE 3–4. A, The hypothetical relationship between inputs to a productive process and the benefits derived describes a production function. As investment continues, the net benefit (ΔB_n) progressively decreases, then becomes negative, illustrating the law of diminishing return. B, Rationalizing rather than rationing healthcare technology achieves maximal benefit at the top of the curve, a level of investment associated with the optimal benefit. Panel A is reproduced with permission from Reference 17. Panel B is modified with permission from References 17 and 18.

issues, is incomplete.[5] The task is complicated further due to our rudimentary understanding of outcomes and economics, which extend well beyond those purely clinical and financial, to include patient functioning, quality of life, patient preferences, and patient-based assessment of care, among other seemingly subjective topics.[19] The problem is not the absence of an appropriate analytic methodology, for cost-effectiveness analysis (CEA)[20–22] is available to aid our decision making (see Chapter 5). Rather, the methodology requires information that we lack: an understanding of the full array of anesthesia-related outcomes, including their incidence under different situations and relationships to other adverse circumstances, and knowledge of patient-based assessments of the outcomes, including preferences for different outcomes and outcome gradations. As a result, CEA is used only occasionally in relation to anesthesia care, and even then in very limited ways (e.g., drug and device cost comparisons), devoid of the patient-derived information and societal perspective that have become an accepted standard.[22]

Even if CEA becomes more commonly used, physicians frequently misunderstand and misuse the underlying concepts, risking incorrect use of the information.[23,24] Patient charges are confused with costs, simplistic quotients of healthcare benefits and costs are invoked in discussions of cost-effectiveness (or worse, cost-benefit), and cost-effectiveness is erroneously equated with cost-savings. Although true CEA *may* guide us to cost-savings, its principal goal is to identify how to obtain the greatest value for what is spent. Although general[21,22,25–33] and anesthesia-specific[4,19,34,35] guidance is available, few anesthesiologists will have sufficient time or expertise to undertake such outcomes-related research. Yet, anesthesiologists must develop an appreciation of the salient considerations when evaluating or planning value-based comparisons of care (Table 3–1).

Marketplace Responses

Far from passive, the purchasers of healthcare services have developed their own approaches to seeking value. Most recently, when proposed national healthcare reform stalled by the mid-1990s, corporate America assumed leadership because healthcare costs had become an increasingly burdensome component of production costs, sapping their business competitiveness internationally. Corporate America sought alternatives to conventional fee-for-service healthcare by quickly shifting increasing numbers of employees into health maintenance organizations and other managed care systems that try to manage the costs, quantity, and quality of healthcare and access to that care. These health plans combine financing and delivery of care, enabling lower health insurance premiums as a result of increased emphasis on preventive services and decreased utilization of specialist physician services. Not satisfied to merely pay lower premiums, however, corporate America has become an active participant

TABLE 3–1. CONSIDERATIONS IN VALUE-BASED COMPARISONS OF CARE

Include economic considerations in clinical decision making: it is neither unethical nor immoral
Be explicit in a comparison; assume nothing: nothing is "obvious"
Identify all possible benefits and risks associated with alternative clinical approaches
Focus on costs, not charges (e.g., patient bills)
Capture indirect costs (e.g., patient's out-of-pocket losses) as well as direct costs
Focus on marginal differences related to alternative approaches, rather than overall cost of care
Emphasize real outcomes (e.g., myocardial infarction) rather than intermediate or surrogate endpoints (e.g., myocardial ischemia) unless they are highly associated
Do not lose sight of implications of early "savings" on even more costly events "downstream" in the care process
Opt for the lower-cost approach unless value is demonstrated in the higher-cost alternative

Modified from Reference 4.

in organizations (e.g., Foundation for Accountability [FACCT], National Committee for Quality Assurance) that are now defining measures of quality of care (e.g., Health Plan Employer Data and Information Set [HEDIS]) and evaluating health plans. In these activities, quality of care is increasingly defined not in technical measures set forth by providers of care, but in ways especially meaningful to consumers of care.

Consumers have also been more active in seeking greater value in healthcare. Despite a recent backlash against managed care's unfettered freedom in restricting or denying access to services, consumers have generally been willing to surrender much of their prerogative to choose providers in trade for lower cost. Yet, consumers are less disposed to passive acceptance of a paternalistic approach to decision making, leading to greater negotiation with their providers. Another patient-related trend has been to supplant the familiar biomedical reductionism, which views the human body as a black box with physiologic processes, with an expanded biopsychosocial model that recognizes not only physiologic processes, but also functional status and quality of life as important considerations. In this more comprehensive model of health, the patient's preferences for and satisfaction with the care provided achieve special importance.

Hence, physicians, health plans, and the settings in which care is delivered are increasingly being pushed to provide care that has greater perceived value and is more patient-centered. Outcomes research provides the perspective and tools to meet these new requirements.

WHAT IS OUTCOMES RESEARCH?

Defining *outcomes research* presents challenges akin to those faced by the blind men in the Indian fable who were asked to describe an elephant based on touching only one part of the large beast. The elephant's stocky legs suggested a tree trunk, and its tail, a snake. Depending on one's perspective, outcomes research may variously appear to be a method to define appropriate care, determine the quality and value of care, or guide the improvement of care, among still other uses. As perhaps expected of a new, emerging field, it crosses the boundaries, borrows, and admixes the methods of related scholarly fields, such as health services research, clinical epidemiology, biostatistics, economics, pharmacoeconomics, informatics, organization theory, and quality improvement. Indeed, outcomes research is like old wine in a new bottle, for the aforementioned studies of appropriateness of care and small-area variations are now considered examples of outcomes research.

Although fraught with imprecision, we may attempt a definition of outcomes research as a comprehensive approach to determining the effects of healthcare using a variety of data sources and measures. It focuses on the *effectiveness of healthcare interventions in customary medical practice* and emphasizes patient benefit at either the individual or aggregate level. Whereas bench laboratory research explores the mechanisms by which an intervention may work, clinical research identifies its potential benefit to the patient (efficacy) and begins to explore the safety of the intervention. Outcomes research completes the research continuum by bridging the gap between what we do and what the intervention actually accomplishes (effectiveness). The goal is to determine *what works in healthcare* and how different providers (practitioners as well as institutions) compare with regard to patient outcomes.

LIMITATIONS OF THE RANDOMIZED CLINICAL TRIAL

At this point, some readers may be wondering, "Doesn't the randomized clinical trial (RCT)—the principal clinical research design long-considered the 'gold standard' in establishing efficacy—establish what works in healthcare?" Unfortunately, the RCT meets this need only to a very limited extent. The RCT's principal strength lies in the randomization process that not only eliminates conscious bias due to physician or patient selection and allocates known patient characteristics (e.g., age, gender) equally between study groups, but also distributes equally between groups unknown factors that may be important in determining intervention outcomes. Because it can control potential sources of bias, the RCT provides the most reliable basis for decision making regarding efficacy, supplanting clinical judgment, which has proven unreliable (Chapter 2 contains a more complete discussion of the importance of the RCT study design).

Nonetheless, the RCT is also problematic.[36] Randomization results in administrative complexity and higher cost and does not guarantee balanced study groups, only groups that are alike on average or equally heterogeneous. There are also ethical issues, the most discussed of which relates to randomly allocating patients to a control group when the intervention is commonly believed to be beneficial, although its efficacy remains to be established in a formal study. More insidious, and undoubtedly much more frequent, is the ethical dilemma posed by randomly allocating patients to study groups when the physician has *some* notion of what is best. In this circumstance, the physician, acting as the physician-*scientist* on behalf of *future* patients, allows a commitment to the present patient to be attenuated, violating assumptions of the physician-patient relationship.[37]

More germane to outcomes research, RCTs typically focus on purely clinical endpoints, which provides only a limited perspective on the value of an intervention and often relates poorly to *customary clinical practice* and the decisions faced by clinicians. There are many explanations for this apparent paradox: RCTs are fairly rigid experiments whose elements are highly selected to enable a definitive result in the most efficient way, thereby avoiding unduly large study populations and related additional expense. Moreover, the subjects have limited or no comorbidity, unlike the unselected patients treated in customary healthcare settings. The comparison intervention may be the standard drug or perhaps a placebo, but the RCT may last so long that newer drugs render the comparator obsolete. We take for granted that subjects randomly allocated to the intervention group actually receive it, administered in the most optimal fashion by highly trained individuals who also monitor the treatment. In contrast, in the real world, patients do not have equal access to care, especially the newest technology, and practitioners may differ in their skill in administering it.

Thus, interventions with equal *efficacy* in an RCT may have different *effectiveness* in the uncontrolled world of customary healthcare. Structure and process in the healthcare system influence whether the intervention's efficacy is manifest as effectiveness. Focusing on the latter, outcomes research is also termed effectiveness research. Table 3–2 summarizes many of the salient differences between outcomes research and conventional clinical research.

TABLE 3–2. COMPARISON OF OUTCOMES RESEARCH AND CONVENTIONAL CLINICAL RESEARCH

	Outcomes Research	Clinical Research
What is studied	Effectiveness	Efficacy
Clinical setting	Customary clinical practice	Ideal clinical practice
Caregivers	Customary personnel	Experienced investigator
Study design(s)	Observational study; randomized, controlled trial (infrequently)	Randomized, controlled trial
Principal measures	Patient-related outcomes[a]	Clinical endpoints
Study subjects	Heterogeneous; usually consecutive	Homogeneous; highly selected
Strength	Relevance to clinical practice	Unbiased proof
Weakness	Possible unknown bias(es)	Limited generalizability

[a]See Table 3 for examples.
Modified after Reference 19.

CHALLENGES POSED BY OBSERVATIONAL STUDIES

With its emphasis on how interventions actually work in customary healthcare settings (effectiveness), outcomes research generally relies on observational studies rather than on RCTs used in conventional clinical research (Table 4–2). Indeed, given their aforementioned limitations, in addition to their high costs and likely infeasibility in many circumstances, RCTs are infrequently used for outcomes studies.[38,39] Instead, outcomes researchers often use an increasing array of data that are accumulated as a by-product of healthcare delivery. This information exists as large databases related to federal programs (e.g., Medicare claims data, National Cancer Institute's Cancer Registry), moderately large databases used for private advocacy (e.g., American Hospital Association's Annual Survey of Hospitals, American Medical Association's Physician Masterfile, American Society of Anesthesiologists [ASA] Closed Claim Study), and smaller data sets created in institutions for a variety of purposes (e.g., billing, resource management, risk management, quality improvement, marketing). Such secondary or administrative data may have a wide variety of outcomes related uses, including studies of the epidemiology of care, impact of policy decisions, quality of care, and costs of care.

Observational data are plagued by a variety of issues and problems that may limit or vitiate their appropriateness for use in a given piece of outcomes research.[40] Because such data were almost always collected for purposes (e.g., bills for services) different from that of one's proposed research, the data elements may be defined differently and generally are of lesser quality, detail, and completeness than that desired for the particular research. Although usually relatively inexpensive to obtain (compared with primary data collection), secondary data may require substantial computer programming expertise to create a usable data set, with resultant large expenditures (e.g., in excess of $50,000 with Medicare claims files).

Use of such secondary data requires thoughtful restraint, particularly a very clear understanding of the limitations inherent in the data set. Are the patient populations and variables in the data truly relevant to the proposed study questions? Might the sampling frame have excluded certain sites and/or patient groups? For example, the ASA Closed Claim Study database contains information on only those patients whose care resulted in a malpractice liability claim, which limits the value of the database to a description of such patients, their injuries, and disposition of their claims. Because the database lacks information on a reference population that underwent anesthesia but did not experience adverse events, the database cannot be explored for risk factors for specific adverse outcomes (the advantages and limitations of this database are discussed in Chapter 8). Is the level of aggregation (e.g., geographic units, services versus episodes of care) appropriate? Is the diagnostic and procedural coding adequate? Problems with these and other technical issues may give rise to (often untreatable) biases that impair the validity of the proposed research.

An especially thorny problem encountered when comparing outcomes in nonrandom, observational studies is that sicker patients are more likely to have worse outcomes. Underlying this truism is the notion that patient outcome is a function of a complex mix of factors, including treatment effectiveness, patient risk factors, quality of care, and random chance variation.[41–43] Clearly, we must incorporate into outcome analysis an adjustment for what we cannot control in the study. Yet, the field of risk adjustment is still very much in its infancy; that there are more than a dozen general-purpose risk-adjustment methods attests to the lack of a fully satisfactory approach.[41–43]

However, anesthesiologists have had the capability to risk adjust their patient outcomes, albeit in a limited way. Although the ASA physical status was intended only as a method to prospectively characterize a patient's preoperative health status,[44] it has been found to be a strong predictor of perioperative death[45–47] and complications.[48,49] Substantial subjectivity in the way that individual practitioners use the classifications[50] limits the precision of the resultant risk adjustment. Yet, when combined with other risk-associated data, the ASA physical status performs rather well: combined with age, type of surgery, and whether the procedure is emergent, the classification accounts for almost all variation in perioperative death rate[47]; combined with age and type of surgery, the classification is highly associated with complication rates and hospital stay.[49]

Clearly, the use of observational data in outcomes research can be as problematic as information learned in RCTs from clinical research. Indeed, the strength of each is the weakness of the other: clinical research provides unbiased proof of efficacy, but its results often have limited generalizability to customary healthcare settings, whereas outcomes research enjoys broad relevance in customary settings, but unknown biases may impair validity (Table 3–2). In the end, we gain confidence in the validity of our conclusions when they are based on research gained from several studies using different approaches and study designs. Although outcomes research and clinical research have been presented herein as separate undertakings—with clinical research focused ultimately on the care of individual patients and outcomes research taking a population-based, societal perspective on healthcare—there is a growing expectation that the two approaches will draw closer, if not eventually come under the same heading. One prominent leader of academic medicine sees an expanded definition of clinical research that would include health services research and the evaluative clinical sciences (e.g., epidemiology, clinical decision analysis, CEA), largely as a result of the training of many clinicians from many disciplines (not restricted to medicine) in the concepts and methods of health services research.[51]

WHAT ARE THE OUTCOMES IN OUTCOMES RESEARCH?

As clinicians, we usually use "outcome" to mean the *clinical* results of care, typically a narrowly defined group of adverse events (e.g., acute myocardial infarction) and even intermediate states (e.g., myocardial ischemia). (Note, too, that we use a highly technical terminology.) However, outcomes researchers use the term much more broadly to convey a comprehensive perspective of an intervention's effectiveness. This use is consistent with the original definition of *outcome:* "a change in a patient's current and future health status that can be attributed to antecedent health care . . . [which includes] social and psychological function in addition to the more usual emphasis on the physical and physiologic aspects of performance."[52] This broader definition of outcome places greater emphasis on the patient perspective, including their preferences, expectations, and assessment of the quality of care. Thus, in addition to clinical outcomes, outcomes research considers three other outcome dimensions: functional status, patient satisfaction, and economic consequences (Table 3–3).

Clinical Outcomes

As active clinicians, anesthesiologists are already very familiar with the spectrum of clinical outcomes, ranging from seemingly minor side effects to major complications and death. Because anesthesia care facilitates other treatment and, with the exception of critical care and pain management, rarely confers independent benefit, our principal focus has been on decreasing the incidence of adverse events, such as postoperative acute myocardial infarction. Because such events occur infrequently, the temptation is to study an intermediate or surrogate event, such as myocardial ischemia, that may be associated with the event of interest but that occurs much more frequently, especially while the patient is under our immediate care. The potential advantages of focusing on a surrogate endpoint include accruing the sample size needed for a study sooner and at a lower cost, because the surrogate event occurs so frequently. However, the countervailing consid-

TABLE 3–3. EXAMPLES OF PATIENT-RELATED OUTCOMES USED IN OUTCOMES RESEARCH

Dimension	Patient-Related Outcomes
Clinical outcomes	Clinical endpoint(s) (symptoms, laboratory values); complications, adverse events; death
Functional health status	Level of function (performance, quality of life): physical, psychologic (well-being), social, role
Patient satisfaction	Patient-based assessment of care: quality, convenience, information, access to care
Economic consequences	Utilization of healthcare resources (tests, drugs, procedures); length of stay (hospital, intensive care unit, office visits); costs (indirect as well as direct); time lost from work (foregone income)

Modified from Reference 19.

eration is how closely associated the occurrence of the surrogate endpoint is with that of the outcome of interest. In this example, myocardial ischemia is often not followed by myocardial infarction;[53] therefore, focusing on ischemia when we are interested in infarction may mislead us. Thus, we must exercise caution in using surrogate endpoints in outcomes research.[2,54]

Functional Status

Consistent with the broad perspective taken in outcomes research, functional status refers not only to the patient's level of physical activity, but also to social and psychological well-being, all of which characterize health-related quality of life (Table 4–3). The latter is a concept that may be characterized by using a wide variety of scales and survey instruments.[29,33,55–63] Whereas some of these scales are disease- or condition-specific, others measure general quality of life; the patient, rather than a healthcare provider, is the respondent. Most of these scales have been validated in a variety of clinical settings, although typically for chronic diseases. Anesthesiologists are beginning to incorporate some of these scales into the longitudinal evaluation of patients with chronic pain,[64] in whom such instruments may be helpful in assessing the value of different interventions. It is incumbent on anesthesiologists to include socially relevant measures in our outcomes research.[65] However, whether these scales can be useful in relation to the transient impairment associated with anesthesia remains to be evaluated.

Patient Satisfaction

More than just whether the patient liked the care and the caregivers, patient satisfaction focuses largely on whether the care was *patient-centered*. Many physicians bristle when hearing this, insisting that what they do is inherently centered on the patient's medical needs. Yet, medical needs are only one subset of a patient's total needs (Table 4–3).

Most patients find modern healthcare confusing, frustrating, and even intimidating. So many healthcare providers may be involved in a given episode of care that the patients may feel as though they are on a conveyor belt, waiting to be processed by a system that functions largely for the convenience of the providers. Who is in charge? As noted earlier, patients also have an increasing desire to have a role in clinical decision making and are eager to express preferences for treatment options, when they exist and there are no overriding clinical considerations. Yet, healthcare providers often do not inquire about such preferences. Thus, assessment of patient satisfaction increasingly considers whether the patient's preferences were elicited and, when appropriate, whether they were incorporated into decision making. Were the patient's (reasonable) expectations met? Were elements of care integrated such that the patient knew who was in charge? At a time when quality is increasingly defined from the customer's perspective (e.g., report cards), such questions are becoming more relevant.[66]

Economic Consequences

Rather than alluding to charges for or even costs of care, economic consequences implies an assessment of the economic burden of the intervention on the patient, the institution at which the care is provided, the healthcare insurer, and—most importantly—society, which ultimately pays for the care. Moreover, instead of merely seeking cost-savings, analyses are increasingly conducted to compare the efficiency of alternative interventions in a search for greater value (at whatever level of spending is chosen) *and* enhanced institutional performance (efficiency). Again, there are many very good sources of general[21,22,25–33] and anesthesia-specific[4,19,34,35] guidance on the economic evaluation of healthcare outcomes and technology.

USING OUTCOMES RESEARCH TO IMPROVE ANESTHESIA CARE

Figure 3–5 presents a framework for considering how outcomes research relates to the many opportunities to enhance quality of care and

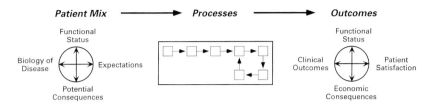

FIGURE 3–5. General schema for improving the value of healthcare using the clinical value compass model. This framework assumes that health is comprised of biological, physical, mental, and social aspects. The aim of healthcare is to reduce or limit the burden of illness by restoring or improving health functioning. Quality healthcare is composed of the care processes most likely to achieve the health outcomes desired by the patient, at a price representing value for that patient. The value of healthcare is a function of quality, costs, and volume. Modified with permission from Reference 66.

improve institutional performance. Not insignificantly, the illustration is based on successful models of quality improvement.[67] Although a discussion of quality improvement is beyond the scope of this chapter, improvement is clearly the terminus in the path that outcomes research charts. Fortunately, there are several excellent sources for guidance.[67–69]

Reducing Inappropriate Variation

Variation abounds in healthcare. Recall the small-area variation studies that have documented substantial variation in the use of resources without commensurate enhancement of outcomes.[13–15] In the absence of an explicit effort to explore alternative approaches, and until proven otherwise, variation should be considered evidence of processes with undue loss, waste, and even poorer outcomes than optimal situations (with little or no variation).

Anesthesiologists have been prominent in identifying variation in outcomes beginning with the mid-century study by Beecher and Todd[70] that documented an unexplained threefold variation in postoperative mortality among study sites. The 1960s National Halothane Studies[71,72] documented a 27-fold variation in postoperative mortality among 34 participating hospitals, which decreased to 3-fold once adjustments were made for patient age, ASA physical status, and type of surgery. Struck by the variation, its principal statisticians urged "quiet, unofficial, cooperatively oriented inquiries," including the exchange of selected members of the staff of two hospitals differing only in death rates, to achieve a better understanding and, possibly, to improve care. "The importance of corrective efforts arises not from their effects (if successful) in these hospitals, but from the benefits which may accrue to wider application of similar efforts later."[73] Exploration into possible explanations for the mortality variations continued in the 1970s Institutional Differences Study, when an investigator involved in the National Halothane Study joined with sociologists to explore nonclinical variables in a national data set.[74,75] Interestingly, they found statistically meaningful (although weak) associations between mortality and variables characterizing the hospital's organizational structure. This study was among the earliest to demonstrate a relationship between performing a high volume of high-risk cases and achieving better outcomes.[75]

Among the best recent examples of how physicians can work together to reduce variation in outcomes and to improve quality of care is the Northern New England Cardiovascular Disease Study Group, comprised of the region's five medical centers performing CABG procedures. Cardiac surgeons representing these sites joined together in the late 1980s to develop a common, shared database describing their practices. With the expert assistance of a clinical epidemiologist, their goal was to use the database to understand and improve their practices. An early product was a multivariable prediction model[76] that they embedded in a chip in a pocket calculator that the cardiac surgeon could use to present patient-specific risk to individual patients. Although not formally studied, a more objective assessment of mortality risk influenced surgical and patient decision making, avoiding high-risk procedures when medical therapy might suffice.[77]

As their database grew, the surgeons met periodically to review the variation in their results, which, in turn, prompted institutional site visits, as suggested more than 20 years earlier in the National Halothane Study,[73] to help them to understand the care processes underlying the observed variation. Hypotheses and related modifications in practice patterns followed in short "tests of change" now encouraged in improvement programs.[67–69] Through iterative improvement cycles, the variation decreased, and the observed mortality decreased 24% from what was expected from the earlier multivariate analysis and national data.[78]

Similar hospital-specific improvement efforts have reported enhanced outcomes in acute myocardial infarction,[79] CABG surgery,[80] and carotid endarterectomy.[81] The recent identification of substantial variation in transfusion practices related to CABG surgery in two dozen sites participating in cooperative data collection[82] highlights yet another opportunity to learn about the determinants of such variation and to develop similar improvement strategies.

Yet another intriguing recent example of how exploring variation in outcomes can improve care relates to critical care medicine, a setting well known for variations in mortality and length of stay.[83,84] Combining statewide discharge data and a survey of intensive care unit (ICU) directors at each hospital, a group of investigators sought to determine whether differences in the organizational characteristics of ICUs were associated with differences in in-hospital mortality and morbidity and in total hospital charges for patients undergoing abdominal aortic surgery.[85] Organizational characteristics associated with increased in-hospital mortality included absence of a full-time ICU medical director, <50% of ICU physicians certified in critical care, not having daily rounds by an ICU physician, and having a decreased ICU nurse to patient ratio in the evening. Critical care certification was also associated with lower hospital charges for these high-risk patients. Decreasing ICU nursing staff below a certain level may lead to increased length of stay and costs of care. The investigators urged consideration of uniform standards for the care of such patients.

Using Technology More Selectively

Outcomes research can also help us to use technology more selectively. Advances in healthcare technology have enhanced our technical capabilities and thereby improved care. However, technology's benefits are achieved only when it is appropriately applied, for the possibility of undesired side effects and complications, as well as increased costs, are associated with its use. Although we may agree on such general tenets, applying them to specific technology is often difficult.

An especially relevant example in cardiovascular medicine is the use of the pulmonary artery catheter. This technology has been used for 25 years in a wide variety of clinical settings, yet its benefit has never been proven in RCTs. Part of the problem in demonstrating its value may lie in the small sample size of those RCTs; however, the sample size required for an adequate RCT is so large (e.g., 20,000 patients to detect a 20% decrease in mortality in CABG surgery) that it is probably not feasible. The task is further complicated by the fact that the catheter itself is not a therapy; its putative value is derived by obtaining unique measurements that may, in turn, guide pharmacotherapy. Especially relevant is the documentation of the widespread gaps in physicians' knowledge related to the use of this technology.[86]

Several years ago, a database was accrued as part of a multicenter study of the preferences and outcomes of severely ill patients whose life expectancy was estimated at about 6 months. More recently, this database was explored with regard to the use of the pulmonary artery catheter.[87] Although the data were collected prospectively, patients could not be randomized to receive or not receive this technology. To treat the obvious bias that sicker patients are more likely to receive the catheter, the investigators used sophisticated multivariate modeling to adjust for this propensity. They found not only that this technology conferred no benefit, but that its use seemed to be associated with worse outcomes. A similar analysis of another observational data set had similar results (Dawson NV, unpublished observations), although a third analysis was indeterminate (Lee TH, unpublished observations).

Nonetheless, many anesthesiologists are convinced that the pulmonary artery catheter is beneficial,[88] even if demonstrating this in a RCT may not be possible. One way to reconcile this situation is to take a different approach using outcomes research. Because no technology is universally beneficial—that is, in some circumstances, not only is there no benefit, but complications may occur—the task is to restrict the use of a given technology to those patients most likely to benefit. From this perspective, the task is to identify a high-risk population for which the catheter offers the greatest potential benefit, then restrict use of the catheter to this population.

The general methodological approach involves development of a clinical prediction rule, essentially a scoring system for prediction of a given outcome based on mathematical modeling of the relative importance of the predictor variables.[89] Familiar examples of clinical prediction rules include Goldman's cardiac risk index,[90] Goldman's stratification protocol to predict acute myocardial infarction in patients presenting to the emergency room with chest pain,[91] and a scoring system for assessing respiratory adequacy after thymectomy via median sternotomy in patients with myasthenia gravis during the preplasmapheresis era.[92]

Investigators in the New England Cardiovascular Disease Study Group are developing the rudiments for a clinical prediction rule for appropriate use of the pulmonary artery catheter in CABG surgery. A critical initial step is defining the outcome to be modeled, which requires identifying specifically what the pulmonary artery catheter is reputed to prevent. Although a variety of adverse outcomes might be chosen, these investigators focused on death, drawing on some of their related analyses.[93] The next step was to identify predictors of the outcome and their relative importance. The investigators found that heart failure was associated with 65% of the deaths, and risk factors for developing fatal heart failure included advanced age, female gender, peripheral vascular disease, prior CABG surgery, and preoperative left ventricular dysfunction. Next, they developed scores for each predictor based on its independent weight in the logistic regression model, and they found that the resultant clinical prediction rule differentiates a high-risk population from other patients who are much less likely to benefit from a pulmonary artery catheter. In a limited application of the rule, catheter use has decreased about 60% without apparent adverse events (O'Connor GT, unpublished observations). Of course, this effort is akin to a trial by exclusion and by no means refutes the value of the catheter. Yet, in a circumstance in which a RCT is probably infeasible, this approach represents a way to decrease arguably inappropriate usage without causing harm.

Achieving Meaningful Cost-Savings

An increasingly competitive healthcare marketplace is placing unprecedented pressure on healthcare practitioners to achieve cost-savings. Clearly, we wish to cut costs, but not if the "savings" are associated with unrecognized but related downstream decrements in quality of care and/or compensatory increases in expenditures. For example, a major initiative in many ICUs is achieving earlier extubation because longer periods of mechanical ventilation are associated with longer stays in the ICU, increased incidence of nosocomial pneumonia, longer hospital stay, and increased hospital cost. These initiatives—commonly characterized as the "fast track," as if there has been an intentional slower track—have involved decreasing the use of long-acting central nervous system depressants and even extubating in the operating room the tracheas of more patients who had been mechanically ventilated in the ICU. Such initiatives make sense only if the patients, many of whom are at high risk of cardiorespiratory complications, actually do well; however, there has been little information on the outcomes of such patients. Particularly worrisome is a recent finding that routinely extubating the tracheas of aortic surgery patients in the operating room was associated with longer length of stay, which suggests increased morbidity.[85]

An application of a more general approach to cost-savings provides insights into clinical economics and valuable guidance.[93] The implementation of an automated anesthetic record, enhanced to include the pharmaceutical agents used in the operating room and care given in the postanesthetic care unit, enabled an anesthesiology department to track its practices and early postanesthetic clinical outcomes. Simultaneously, the department developed pharmaceutical practice guidelines, emphasizing especially costly drugs, that were based on published literature on drug effects and actual hospital costs. They also conducted various educational initiatives to foster acceptance of the new guidelines and adoption of cost-saving practice patterns. Successful implementation of the guidelines enabled substantial savings without apparent decrement in early postanesthetic clinical outcomes. This effort is a model for a physician-led approach that should be fostered in all clinical settings (this work is described in Chapter 5).

Meeting Patient Preferences

Patients are increasingly interested in greater involvement in clinical decision making related to their care,[95] and quality of care is increasingly evaluated from the patient's perspective. As a result, we should make a greater effort to develop care that is more patient-centered whenever possible. Unfortunately, despite a rich literature on complications and side effects related to anesthesia care, there is little information on what patients want and value in their care.

Emerging in this scant literature is that patients' perspectives, although individual, may have common themes. Emetic symptoms are especially troublesome, and, significantly, the economic value placed on avoidance of these symptoms equates with the costs of prophylaxis.[96] Acute postoperative pain continues to be a focus of patients' concern,[97] despite the availability of enhanced technology for its treatment[98,99] and the increasing importance of such experiences in patients' assessment of the care. Learning about and finding ways to meet patients' preferences for care is especially fertile ground for outcomes research.

References

1. Lee A, Lum ME: Measuring anaesthetic outcomes. Anaesth Intensive Care 24:685–693, 1996
2. Wedel DJ, Brennan TJ, White PF, Sandler A: Workshop on how to perform clinical outcome studies. Anesthesiology 87:1021–1022, 1997
3. Lee PR, Soffel D, Luft HS: Costs and coverage: Pressures toward health care reform. West J Med 157:576–583, 1992
4. Orkin FK: Moving toward value-based anesthesia care. J Clin Anesth 5:91–98, 1993
5. Naylor CD: What is appropriate care? N Engl J Med 338:1918–1921, 1998
6. Brook RH, Chassin MR, Fink A, Solomon DH, Kosecoff J, Park RE: A method for the detailed assessment of the appropriateness of medical technologies. Int J Technol Assess Health Care 2:56–63, 1986
7. Park RE, Fink A, Brook RH, Chassin MR, Kahn KL, Merrick NJ, Kosecoff J, Solomon DH: Physician ratings of appropriate indications for six medical and surgical procedures. Am J Pub Health 76:766–772, 1986
8. Leape LL, Hilborne LH, Park RH, Bernstein SJ, Kamberg CJ, Sherwood M, Brook RH: The appropriateness of use of coronary artery bypass graft surgery in New York State. JAMA 269:753–760, 1993
9. Office of Technology Assessment, United States Congress: Strategies for Medical Technology Assessment, p. 3, United States Government Printing Office, 1982
10. Shekelle PG, Kahan JP, Bernstein SJ, Leape LL, Kamberg CJ, Park RE: The reproducibility of a method to identify the overuse and underuse of medical procedures. N Engl J Med 338:1888–1895, 1998
11. Ayanian JZ, Landrum MB, Normand S-LT, Guadagnoli E, McNeil

BJ: Rating the appropriateness of coronary arteriography: Do practicing physicians agree with an expert panel and with each other? N Engl J Med 338:1896–1904, 1998
12. Wennberg JE, Gittelsohn A: Small area variations in health care delivery: A population-based health information system can guide planning and regulatory decision-making. Science 182:1102–1108, 1973
13. Wennberg JE, Gittelsohn A: Variations in medical care among small areas. Sci Am 246:120–134, 1982
14. Wennberg JE, Freeman JL, Shelton RM, Bubolz TA: Hospital use and mortality among Medicare beneficiaries in Boston and New Haven. N Engl J Med 321:1168–1173, 1989
15. Wennberg JE, Cooper MM (eds): The Dartmouth Atlas of Health Care 1998. Chicago, American Hospital Publishing, 1998
16. Wennberg JE: Incidence of surgery, case fatality rate and probability of death from surgery among populations. In Hirsh RA, Forrest WH, Orkin FK, Wollman H (eds): Health Care Delivery in Anesthesia, pp. 41–47. Philadelphia, George F. Stickley, 1980
17. Orkin FK: Patient monitoring during anesthesia as an exercise in technology assessment. In Saidman LJ, Smith NT (eds): Monitoring in Anesthesia, (3rd ed), pp. 439–455, Stoneham, MA, Butterworth-Heinemann, 1993
18. Reinhardt UE: The importance of quality in the debate on national health policy. In Couch JB (ed): Health Care Quality Management for the 21st Century, pp. 1–22. Tampa, FL, American College of Physician Executives, 1991
19. Orkin FK: Outcomes research in anesthesia. Adv Anesth 16:99–128, 1999.
20. Weinstein MC, Stason WB: Foundations of cost-effectiveness analysis for health and medical practices. N Engl J Med 296:716–721, 1977
21. Weinstein MC, Fineberg HC (eds): Clinical Decision Analysis. Philadelphia, WB Saunders, 1980
22. Gold MR, Siegel JE, Russell LB, Weinstein MC (eds): Cost-Effectiveness in Health and Medicine. New York, Oxford University Press, 1996
23. Doubilet P, Weinstein MC, McNeil BJ: Use and misuse of the term "cost effective" in medicine. N Engl J Med 314:253–255, 1986
24. Udvarhelyi IS, Colditz GA, Rai A, Epstein AM: Cost-effectiveness and cost-benefit analyses in the medical literature: Are the methods being used correctly? Ann Intern Med 116:238–244, 1992
25. Eisenberg JM: Clinical economics: A guide to the economic analysis of clinical practices. JAMA 262:2879–2886, 1989
26. Detsky AS, Naglie IG: A clinician's guide to cost-effectiveness analysis. Ann Intern Med 113:147–154, 1990

27. Luce BR, Elixhauser A: Standards for Socioeconomic Evaluation of Health Care Products and Services. Springer-Verlag, 1990
28. Bootman JL, Townsend RJ, McGhan WF (eds): Principles of Pharmacoeconomics (2nd ed). Harvey Whitney Books, 1996
29. Spilker B (ed): Quality of Life and Pharmacoeconomics in Clinical Trials (2nd ed). Philadelphia, Lippincott-Raven, 1996
30. Drummond MF, O'Brien B, Stoddart GL, Torrance GW: Methods for the Economic Evaluation of Health Care Programmes (2nd ed). New York, Oxford Medical, 1997
31. Canadian Coordinating Office for Health Technology Assessment: Guidelines for Economic Evaluation of Pharmaceuticals: Canada (2nd ed). Canadian Coordinating Office for Health Technology Assessment, 1997
32. Drummond MF, Richardson WS, O'Brien BJ, Levine M, Heyland D: User's guide to the medical literature. XIII. How to use an article on economic analysis of clinical practice. A. Are the results of the study valid? JAMA 277:1552–1557, 1997
33. Cramer JA, Spilker B: Quality of Life & Pharmacoeconomics: An Introduction. Philadelphia, Lippincott-Raven, 1998
34. Sperry RJ: Principles of economic analysis. Anesthesiology 86:1197–1205, 1997
35. Watcha MF, White PF: Economics of anesthetic practice. Anesthesiology 86:1170–1196, 1997
36. Feinstein AR: An additional basic science for clinical medicine. II. The limitations of randomized trials. Ann Intern Med 99:544–550, 1983
37. Hellman S, Hellman DS: Of mice but not men: Problems of the randomized clinical trial. N Engl J Med 324:1585–1589, 1991
38. Block PC, Ockene I, Goldberg RJ, Butterly J, Block EH, Degon C, Beiser A, Colton T: A prospective randomized trial of outpatient cardiac catheterization. N Engl J Med 319:1251–1255, 1988
39. Brook RH, Ware JE, Rogers WH, et al: Does free care improve adults' health? Results from a randomized controlled trial. N Engl J Med 309:1426–1434, 1983
40. Connell FA, Diehr P, Hart LG: The use of large data bases in health care studies. Ann Rev Public Health 8:51–74, 1987
41. Iezzoni LI: Risk adjustment for medical effectiveness research: An overview of conceptual and methodological considerations. J Invest Med 43:136–150, 1995
42. Iezzoni LI: The risks of risk adjustment. JAMA 278:1600–1607, 1997
43. Iezzoni LI (ed): Risk Adjustment for Measuring Health Outcomes (2nd ed). Ann Arbor, MI, Health Administration Press, 1997
44. Saklad M: Grading of patients for surgical procedures. Anesthesiology 2:281–284, 1941

45. Vacanti CJ, Van Houten RJ, Hill RC: A statistical analysis of the relationship of physical status to postoperative mortality in 68,388 cases. Anesth Analg 49:564–566, 1970
46. Marx GF, Mateo CV, Orkin LR: Computer analysis of post anesthetic death. Anesthesiology 39:54–58, 1973
47. Cohen MM, Duncan PG, Tate RB: Does anesthesia contribute to operative mortality? JAMA 260:2859–2861, 1988
48. Cohen MM, Duncan PG: Physical status score and trends in anaesthetic complications. J Clin Epidemiol 41:83–90, 1988
49. Cullen DJ, Apolone G, Greenfield S, Guadagnoli E, Cleary PD: ASA physical status and age predict morbidity after three surgical procedures. Ann Surg 220:3–9, 1994
50. Owens WD, Felts JA, Spitznagel EL Jr: ASA physical status classification: A study of consistency of ratings. Anesthesiology 49:239–243, 1978
51. Shine KI: President's report to the Institute of Medicine: The health sciences, health services research, and the role of the health professions. Health Serv Res 33:439–445, 1998
52. Donabedian A: Evaluating the quality of medical care. Milbank Mem Fund Q 44(Part 2):166–206, 1966
53. Slogoff S, Keats AS: Does perioperative myocardial ischemia lead to postoperative myocardial infarction? Anesthesiology 62:107–114, 1985
54. Fisher DM: Surrogate end points: Are they meaningful? Anesthesiology 81:795–796, 1994
55. Guyatt GH, Feeney DH, Patrick DL: Measuring health-related quality of life. Ann Intern Med 118:622–629, 1993
56. Wilson IB, Cleary PD: Linking clinical variables with health-related quality of life: A conceptual model of patient outcomes. JAMA 273:59–65, 1995
57. Testa MA, Simonson DC: Assessment of quality-of-life outcomes. N Engl J Med 334:835–840, 1996
58. Bowling A: Measuring Disease: A Review of Disease-Specific Quality of Life Measurement Scales. Bristol, PA, Open University Press, 1995
59. Stewart AL, Ware JE Jr (eds): Measuring Functioning and Well-Being: The Medical Outcomes Study Approach. Durham, NC, Duke University Press, 1996
60. McDowell I, Newell C: Measuring Health: A Guide to Rating Scales and Questionnaires (2nd ed). New York, Oxford University Press, 1996
61. Bowling A: Measuring Health: A Review of Quality of Life Measurement Scales (2nd ed). Bristol, PA, Open University Press, 1997

62. Frank-Stromborg M, Olsen SJ (eds): Instruments for Clinical Health Care Research (2nd ed). Sudbury, MA, Jones & Bartlett, 1997
63. Staquet MJ, Hays RD, Fayers PM: Quality of Life Assessment in Clinical Trials: Methods and Practice. New York, Oxford University Press, 1998
64. Lee VC, Rowlingson JC: Defining quality of life in chronic pain. In Spilker B (ed): Quality of Life and Pharmacoeconomics in Clinical Trials (2nd ed), pp. 853–864. Philadelphia, Lippincott-Raven, 1996
65. Orkin FK, Cohen MM, Duncan PG: The quest for meaningful outcomes. Anesthesiology 78:417–422, 1993
66. Lathrop JP: Restructuring Health Care: The Patient-Focused Paradigm. San Francisco, Jossey-Bass, 1993
67. Nelson EC, Batalden PB, Ryer JC (eds): Clinical Improvement Action Guide. Oakbrook Terrace, IL, Joint Commission on Accreditation of Healthcare Organizations, 1998
68. Langely GJ, Nolan KM, Nolan TW, Norman CL, Provost LP: The Improvement Guide: A Practical Approach to Enhancing Organizational Performance. San Francisco, Jossey-Bass, 1996
69. Berwick DM: A primer on leading the improvement of systems. BMJ 312:619–622, 1996
70. Beecher HK, Todd DP: A study of the deaths associated with anesthesia and surgery. Ann Surg 140:2–34, 1954
71. Subcommittee on the National Halothane Study of the Committee on Anesthesia, National Academy of Sciences, National Research Council: Summary of the National Halothane Study. JAMA 197:775–789, 1966
72. Bunker JP, Forrest WH Jr, Mosteller F, Vandam LD: The National Halothane Study: A Study of the Possible Association Between Halothane Anesthesia and Postoperative Hepatic Necrosis. National Academy of Sciences, National Research Council, 1969
73. Moses LE, Mosteller F: Institutional differences in postoperative death rates: Commentary on some of the findings of the National Halothane Study. JAMA 203:492–493, 1968
74. Scott WR, Forrest WH Jr, Brown BW: Hospital structure and postoperative mortality and morbidity. In Shortell SM, Brown M (eds): Organizational Research in Hospitals, pp. 72–89. Chicago, Inquiry (Blue Cross Association), 1976
75. Flood AB, Scott WR (eds): Hospital Structure and Performance. Baltimore, Johns Hopkins University Press, 1987
76. O'Connor GT, Plume SK, Olmstead EM, Coffin LH, Morton JR, Maloney CT, Nowicki ER, Levy DG, Tryzelaar JF, Hernandez F, Adrian L, Casey KJ, Bundy D, Soule DN, Marrin CAS, Nugent WC, Charlesworth DC, Clough R, Katz S, Leavitt BJ, Wennberg JE: Mul-

tivariate prediction of in-hospital mortality associated with coronary artery bypass graft surgery. Circulation 85:2110–2118, 1992
77. Nugent WC, Schults WC: Playing by the numbers: How collecting outcomes data changed my life. Ann Thorac Surg 58:1866–1870, 1994
78. O'Connor GT, Plume SK, Olmstead EM, Morton JR, Maloney CT, Nugent WC, Hernandez F Jr, Clough R, Leavitt BJ, Coffin LH, Marrin CAS, Wennberg D, Birkmeyer JD, Charlesworth DC, Malenka DJ, Quinton HB, Kasper JF: A regional intervention to improve the hospital mortality associated with coronary artery bypass surgery: The Northern New England Cardiovascular Disease Study Group. JAMA 275:841–846, 1996
79. Nelson EC, Greenfield S, Hays RD, Larson C, Leopold B, Batalden PB: Comparing outcomes and charges for patients with acute myocardial infarction in three community hospitals: An approach for assessing "value." Int J Qual Health Care 7:98–108, 1995
80. Turley K, Turley KM: Reducing length of stay and improving outcomes. In Spath PL (ed): Beyond Clinical Paths: Advanced Tools for Outcomes Management, pp. 163–178. Chicago, American Hospital Publishing, 1997
81. Schneider JR, Droste JS, Golan JF: Impact of carotid endarterectomy critical pathway on surgical outcome and hospital stay. Vasc Surg 31:685–690, 1997
82. Stover EP, Siegel LC, Parks R, Levin J, Body SC, Maddi R, D'Ambra MN, Mangano DT: Variability in transfusion practice for coronary artery bypass surgery persists despite national consensus guidelines. Anesthesiology 88:327–333, 1998
83. Knaus WA, Draper EA, Wagner DP, Zimmerman JE: An evaluation of outcome from intensive care in major medical centers. Ann Intern Med 104:410–418, 1986
84. Knaus WA, Wagner DP, Zimmerman JE, Draper EA: Variations in hospital mortality and length of stay from intensive care. Ann Intern Med 118:753–761, 1993
85. Provonost P, Dorman T, Jenckes M, Garrett E, Breslow M, Rosenfeld B, Lipsett P, Bass E: Organizational characteristics of intensive care units related to outcomes of abdominal aortic surgery. JAMA In press.
86. Iberti TJ, Fischer EP, Leibowitz AB, Panacek EA, Silverstein JH, Albertson TE: A multicenter study of physicians' knowledge of the pulmonary artery catheter. JAMA 264:2928–2932, 1990
87. Connors AF Jr, Speroff T, Dawson NV, Thomas C, Harrell FE Jr, Wagner D, Desbiens N, Goldman L, Wu AW, Califf RM, Fulkerson WJ Jr, Vidaillet H, Broste S, Bellamy P, Lynn J, Knaus WA: The effectiveness of right heart catheterization in the initial care of critically ill patients. JAMA 276:889–897, 1996

88. Tuman KJ, Roizen MF: Outcome assessment and pulmonary artery catheterization: Why does the debate continue? Anesth Analg 84:1–4, 1997
89. Wasson JH, Sox HC, Neff RK, Goldman L: Clinical prediction rules: Applications and methodologic standards. N Engl J Med 313:793–799, 1985
90. Goldman L, Caldera DL, Nussbaum SR, Southwick FS, Krogstad D, Murray B, Burke DS, O'Malley TA, Goroll AH, Caplan CH, Nolan J, Carabello B, Slater EE: Multifactorial index of cardiac risk in noncardiac surgical procedures. N Engl J Med 297:845–850, 1977
91. Goldman L, Cook EF, Brand DA, Lee TH, Rouan GW, Weisberg MC, Acampora D, Stasiulewicz C, Walshon J, Terranova G, Gottlieb L, Kobernick M, Goldstein-Wayne B, Copen D, Daley K, Brandt AA, Jones D, Mellors J, Jakubowski R: A computer protocol to predict myocardial infarction in emergency department patients with chest pain. N Engl J Med 318:797–803, 1988
92. Leventhal SR, Orkin FK, Hirsh RA: Prediction of the need for postoperative mechanical ventilation in myasthenia gravis. Anesthesiology 53:26–30, 1980
93. O'Connor GT, Birkmeyer JD, Dacey LJ, Quinton H, Marrin CAS, O'Connor Birkmeyer N, Morton JR, Leavitt BJ, Maloney CT, Hernandez F Jr, Clough R, Nugent WC, Olmstead EM, Charlesworth DC, Plume SK: Results of a regional study of modes of death associated with coronary artery bypass grafting. Circulation in press.
94. Lubarksy DA, Glass PSA, Ginsberg B, Dear GdeL, Dentz ME, Gan TJ, Sanderson IC, Mythen MG, Dufore S, Pressley CC, Gilbert WC, White WD, Alexander ML, Coleman RL, Rogers M, Reves JG: The successful implementation of pharmaceutical practice guidelines: Analysis of associated outcomes and cost savings. Anesthesiology 86:1145–1160, 1997
95. Barry MJ, Cherkin DC, Chang Y-C, Fowler FJ, Skates S: A randomized trial of a multimedia shared decision-making program for men facing a treatment decision for benign prostatic hyperplasia. Dis Manage Clin Outcomes 1:5–14, 1997
96. Orkin FK: Preferences and willingness-to-pay for postanesthetic recovery states. Med Dec Making 17:543, 1997
97. Lynch EP, Lazor MA, Gellis JE, Orav J, Goldman L, Marcantonio ER: Patient experience of pain after elective noncardiac surgery. Anesth Analg 85:117–123, 1997
98. Treat the pain. Wall Street Journal, July 27, 1998, p A14
99. Walker JD: Enhancing patient comfort. In Gerteis M, Edgman-Levitan S, Daley J, Delbanco TL (eds): Through the Patient's Eyes: Understanding and Promoting Patient-Centered Care, pp. 119–153. San Francisco, Jossey-Bass, 1993

Barbara E. Tardiff
James G. Jollis
David A. Lubarsky

4 | The Use of Information Systems and Large Databases in Cardiovascular Medicine

Information systems play a fundamental role in clinical practice. By bringing order to the chaos of data accrued in the process of medical care, we can better apply our experience to manage patients and systems. The goal of this chapter is to provide a rationale for a systematic process for data collection and retrieval within a healthcare system. Clinical information systems can help to improve the care of the patients by 1) capturing more reliable information; 2) transferring information more effectively, both cost- and time-wise, among healthcare providers; and 3) providing a systematic context for dealing with decisions in clinical care, finances, and quality assurance.

THE CLINICAL INFORMATION SYSTEM

There are three key issues that should be defined in the specification of a clinical database management system:[1-2] 1) the focus of the database—that is, what aspects of the patient's experience are to be captured?; 2) the function of the database—what it will accomplish for the healthcare team; and 3) the form of the database—how it is designed to achieve the defined goals. Like good designs in other domains, form should follow function.

Outcome Measurements, edited by Kenneth Tuman. Lippincott Williams & Wilkins, Baltimore © 1999

Focus

The focus of the database is usually defined by the intended analyses. Analyses tend to fall into one of two general categories: process measurements and outcome assessments. Process measurements incorporate evaluation of the content of care. Outcomes of interest may include clinical, economic, or functional (quality of life) endpoints. The only difference between these two categories involves "compared to what." Outcome assessment is much more difficult than process measurement. It requires a large number of patients and events to derive a stable estimate and sufficient data to risk-adjust; the results do not necessarily indicate how to improve the care or outcome.

The focus of a cardiovascular database may be as simple as record keeping before and after a procedure. However, it is often desirable to link procedural data to other data, including other procedures and other aspects of the clinical course. The scope of a database may also be expanded to include complication data or more complex historic information. If the complete course of a patient is desired, this may require linking procedural databases with inpatient and outpatient records. Each level of expansion of focus involves greater complexity and commitment of resources.

Function

Typical information system functions fall into one of several categories based on what the system is to accomplish.[3] Examples of limited clinical functions include computerized reports to replace dictated or handwritten reports or an electronic depiction of specialized data, such as a map of the coronary arteries. Systems that capture broad clinical functions may support multiple domains or provide for a longitudinal, computerized patient record. Common administrative functions include billing, scheduling, and inventory management. When linked with clinical data, these administrative data can be used to support clinical activities. For example, quality assurance information can be provided for credentialing; computerized inventory systems may be leveraged to provide a complete procedure report. Other systems support medical research.

Form

The form of the database and information management system should be based on the type of data to be collected, the clinical environment for collection; the methods of data entry, storage, and retrieval; the need for flexibility; and the capabilities for analysis. It is critical to consider workflow, as well as technical constraints. The ultimate choice should reflect an evaluation of the various tradeoffs.

In clinical reporting, the view of the patient is a paramount consideration in determining form.[3] For patients with cardiovascular disease undergoing an evaluation or procedure, the likelihood of further cardiovascular evaluation and intervention is very high. Patients with cardiovascular disease also often require a multifaceted approach to the medical problem, and, in many cases, different physicians may provide different aspects of care. In these cases, integration of information from multiple sources provides the basis on which decisions can be made. This need for integration underscores the needs for a common nomenclature and for standard data formats that are readily transferable, not only throughout the hospital, but across geographic regions.

Characteristics of the healthcare system and its complexity place additional requirements on the design of the information system. Points to consider when designing or selecting an information system include the geographic distribution of the network of involved physicians, agreements or relationships beyond the doctor-patient relationship that may affect the pattern of care, and the economics of the system.

USING THE DATA

Regardless of the focus, intended function, or form, a common thread of clinical information systems is that they allow patient information to be collected and stored in a database to be recalled for future use or reference. The cumulative content of these databases provides a fertile ground for building new knowledge and improving medical care. The following discussion provides an overview of cardiovascular research using large databases. It also provides selected examples of how various types of questions about patient outcome and clinician performance have been approached using clinical and administrative databases.

Databases are typically classified according to their original intended purpose. Population databases record vital statistics of individuals in a population and include the census and vital records. Administrative databases are typically assembled for organizing or financing the delivery of health services. Medicare claims data and quality assurance data are administrative databases often exploited to support evaluations of clinical care. Disease registries are compiled by professional societies, such as the American College of Cardiology, the American Heart Association, or the Society of Thoracic Surgeons, or other stakeholders involved in treating patients with a particular disease. Other databases can be assembled in the process of completing a randomized clinical trial. Clinical databases are created for use in the delivery of care and medical records.

Research using large databases, irrespective of their original intended purpose, has several real strengths. Large sample sizes may be accrued. Patients are not selected and often represent many institutions with wide geographic spreads. There is therefore an approximation of a universe of experience. Longitudinal records provide documentation of the natural history of disease and track patient, physician, and hospital identifiers that may be relevant to the evaluation. It is usually possible to closely define the sampling time frame. Finally, it is efficient to use data already collected for another purpose, be it clinical, administrative, or randomized clinical trial. In the best cases, data collection is unobtrusive, systematic, and computer-based.

Evaluation of observational databases is particularly valuable in circumstances in which a randomized clinical trial is unlikely, such as when a therapy is already accepted as effective, when physician support is lacking for an alternative approach, when randomization is difficult, or when financial incentives are limited.

Perhaps the most important feature of large databases is that they permit evaluation of actual practice. To understand how information systems can be used to support clinical decision-making, it is important to differentiate efficacy from effectiveness. Questions of efficacy really can be answered only through controlled clinical trials. However, the downside of the experimental setting is that the result is often obtained in ideal circumstances; that is, in a narrowly defined population receiving optimal care. The quantification of effectiveness answers a somewhat different question—how a treatment works in general use, in unselected patients, and at unselected institutions.

Observational databases occupy a niche in the spectrum of clinical research different from that served by randomized controlled trials. Databases are characteristically well suited for the evaluation of prognosis and predictors of various types of outcomes—clinical, economical, and functional. Recently, there has been emphasis on process measurement, looking at practice patterns and the cost and outcomes of medical care. Contracts go to those with the lowest prices. Profits go to those who are most efficient. Lacking adequate data, healthcare is currently price/large purchase-dominated rather than efficiency (quality for the lowest price)-dominated.

Process Measurement

A large, important area of clinical research activity using databases is process measurement. Processes are easier to measure than outcomes.

The sample sizes needed are smaller, and risk adjustment is not necessary. In addition, it is much easier to interpret and apply the results to improve care.

Databases can play a valuable role in quality assurance in medical care. Although there are limitations and the potential for abuse of these data, they are useful in comparing actual practice with standards of practice, and, in that way, they prompt hospitals and physicians to examine the care they provide. Physicians will increasingly need to justify their clinical decisions based on patient outcomes and cost. For critically ill patients, the necessary adjustments for severity of illness can be made only with a sophisticated computer system.

As an example, Medicare provides hospital-specific reports on mortality for specific diagnoses. Certain healthcare systems (Veterans Affairs, the State of New York) collect hospital-based morbidity and mortality reports to investigate outliers to determine whether standards are met by practitioners. Increasingly, business consortia are collecting data on hospitals to help to recommend referrals for their employees.

Another example of this type of work is that of the Cooperative Cardiovascular Project. This represents a collaboration composed of peer-review organizations in Alabama, Iowa, Wisconsin, and Connecticut, that collects and analyzes detailed clinical data on patients with acute myocardial infarction. The data presented herein are for patients treated between July and December 1992.

Figure 4–1 shows the proportion of patients treated with selected medical therapies for which there is strong evidence of a benefit for patients with acute myocardial infarction.[4] Although a substantial majority of eligible patients were treated with aspirin, rates are significantly

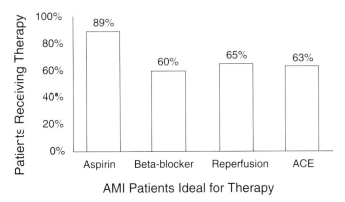

FIGURE 4–1. Evidence-based use of selected medical therapies in patients with acute myocardial infarction (AMI).[4] ACE, angiotensin-converting enzyme inhibitors.

lower for other proven therapies. Figure 4–2 depicts the risk-adjusted mortality rates and 95% confidence intervals for patients with an acute myocardial infarction admitted to various hospitals. Mortality varied substantially among these institutions.[5]

Jollis et al.[6] performed a similar analysis of health policy in the elderly population using Medicare claims data. The population for these analyses included all patients with a discharge diagnosis of acute myocardial infarction or a complication of acute myocardial infarction in 1992. The use of aspirin, β-blockers, and thrombolytics differed significantly by specialty in this population (Figure 4–3). Figure 4–4 illustrates procedure use by specialty.[7] Again, there were significant differences in

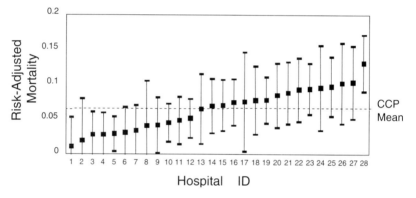

FIGURE 4–2. Risk-adjusted mortality rates and 95% confidence intervals for patients with acute myocardial infarction, by institution.[5] The horizontal dashed line is the mean risk-adjusted mortality for the Cooperative Cardiovascular Project (CCP).

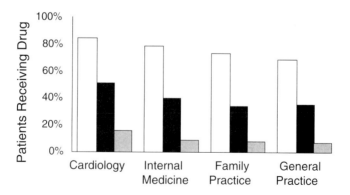

FIGURE 4–3. Use of aspirin (□), β-blockers (■), and thrombolytic therapy (■) in patients with acute myocardial infarction by physician specialty.[6]

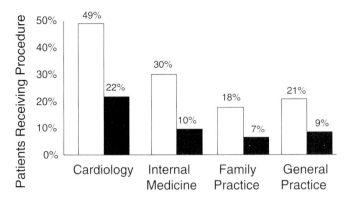

FIGURE 4–4. Use of angiography (□) and angioplasty or bypass surgery (■) in patients with acute myocardial infarction by physician specialty.[7]

the use of catheterizations and revascularization procedures by specialty. There were also mortality differences by specialty (Figure 4–5).[8] These types of data provide valuable descriptions of the outcomes of care at different institutions and by different providers. It is often much more difficult to determine why these differences occur.

Outcomes Assessment

Gathering useful information for outcomes assessment is more difficult. In addition to collecting outcomes, it is necessary to collect the factors that predict outcome and data that measure treatments. Large numbers of patients must be evaluated to obtain stable estimates. Even with good data, it is often difficult to know what to do to improve care based on the information. It is often impossible to determine the reasons for mortality, outcome, or process differences versus differences in illness severity.

Still, large databases that capture detailed clinical data can be extremely useful in evaluating the clinical, functional, and economic impact of individual diseases and practices. Percutaneous versus surgical revascularization is a familiar treatment comparison. Table 4–1 shows the number of patients enrolled in six randomized clinical trials evaluating angioplasty versus bypass surgery.[9–14] The number of patients enrolled in these trials represented only a small fraction of the patients eligible at the participating institutions (4%–17%). These studies may therefore be limited by the selection criteria used to control patient entry, including the selection of participating sites, and the results may not be representative of the community at large.

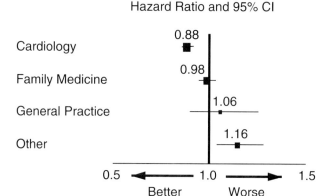

FIGURE 4–5. Mortality at 1 year in patients with acute myocardial infarction by physician specialty and after adjustment for patient and hospital characteristics.[8]

TABLE 4–1. PATIENTS ENROLLED IN SIX RANDOMIZED CLINICAL TRIALS OF ANGIOPLASTY VERSUS BYPASS SURGERY

Study	n	Median Age (yr)	Enrolled (%)	Median Follow-Up (yr)
GABI (8)	358	59	4	1
RITA (9)	1011	57	5	3
EAST (10)	392	62	8	3
ERACI (11)	127	57	17	3
CABRI (12)	1054	60	5	1
BARI (15)	1829	61	7	5

To contrast efficacy with effectiveness in evaluating angioplasty and bypass surgery for patients with symptomatic, ischemic heart disease, it is interesting to contrast data obtained from the Duke Databank for Cardiovascular Disease[15] and data from the Bypass Angioplasty Revascularization Investigation (BARI) trial.[16] The Duke Databank began in 1969 and was designed as a research tool integrated with clinical practice. All angiography, angioplasty, and bypass surgery procedures, as well as various functional tests and clinical progress notes, are incorporated into the medical record through this system. More than 25,000 patients are followed longitudinally with annual follow-ups. Patients in the Duke cohort were selected from those treated between March 1984 and August 1990. The final study population consisted of 3,220 patients with symptomatic coronary artery disease amenable to either procedure. The mean follow-up for this population was 62 years.

Table 4–2 shows a comparison of baseline characteristics between patients in these two analyses. The Duke cohort was slightly older, had more hypertension, higher incidences of prior myocardial infarction and heart failure, more severe coronary disease, and a lower ejection fraction. After adjustment for differences in baseline characteristics between the two populations, 5-year mortality was compared, stratified by the presence of diabetes (Figure 4–6). Survival in diabetics was consistently lower than that in the nondiabetic population. However, in contrast to the BARI results, the difference in survival between diabetics and nondiabetics in the Duke population appears to be similar in both angioplasty-treated and bypass-treated patients in both the adjusted and unadjusted models. Thus, when applied to a general population of diabetic patients (effectiveness), both treatment strategies ap-

TABLE 4–2. BASELINE CHARACTERISTICS OF PATIENTS IN THE DUKE DATABANK AND IN THE BARI POPULATION

	Duke (14) ($n = 3220$)	BARI (15) ($n = 1829$)
Age	63	61.5
Male sex (%)	75	73
Hypertension (%)	54	49
Previous myocardial infarction (%)	60	55
Previous congestive heart failure (%)	11	9
Ejection fraction	52	59
Three-vessel disease (%)	53	41

Values are median or %.

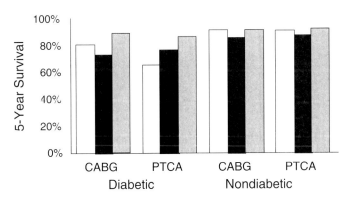

FIGURE 4–6. Stratified 5-year survival in the BARI trial (□) compared with the 5-year unadjusted (■) and adjusted survival (■) in the Duke population.[14,15] CABG, coronary artery bypass surgery; PTCA, percutaneous transluminal coronary angioplasty.

pear equivalent, possibly due to the higher level of illness in the diabetic cohort, which negates the survival benefit for bypass surgery observed in the randomized trials (efficacy).

One of the limitations of databases such as the Duke Databank and other clinical databases is that they typically represent only a single or few centers of experience. An exception is the Global Utilization of Streptokinase and TPA (alteplase) for Occluded Coronary Arteries database, which includes data from more than 40,000 patients from 15 countries around the world. Table 4–3 lists some of the clinical features of patients with acute myocardial infarction that have been explored in this database. The data in clinical trial databases are often among the most reliable because they are subject to numerous data-integrity checks. However, unless they were specifically designed to answer the secondary questions, they are still subject to the same limitations of other clinical data. These databases can also be extremely useful for documenting the clinical features and natural history of a disease.

CURRENT ISSUES

Large databases derived from administrative, clinical, and research information systems can clearly be very useful tools to support decision-making in the delivery and management of cardiovascular healthcare. Although there are important issues related to data collection and statistical methods, information technology is no longer a major limitation, and statistical methods have matured to a stable point. The greatest deficiency is in reliable, quality information. We collect much information in the process of care, but much of it is unstructured (free text), incon-

TABLE 4–3. CLINICAL FEATURES OF PATIENTS WITH ACUTE MYOCARDIAL INFARCTION EXPLORED IN THE GUSTO-I DATABASE[a]

Time to thrombolysis	Heparin dosing
Regional variations in resource use	Non–Q-wave infarction
TIMI flow versus outcome	ST-segment monitoring
Cardiogenic shock	Diabetes
Troponin	Quality of life
Bleeding	Age
Stroke	Sex
Invasive care	Early discharge
Left bundle branch block	ST-segment depression
Menstruation	Atrial fibrillation
Predicting mortality	Pulse variability

TIMI, thrombolysis in myocardial infarction.
[a]The GUSTO Investigators. An international randomized trial comparing four thrombolytic strategies for acute myocardial infarction. N Engl J Med 329:673–682, 1993.

sistently collected, or poorly defined. Structured data and standard definitions may create a less personal medical record, but they provide more information that can be used to improve clinical care.

Data Collection

While technological advances have made the management of large databases much easier than it was a few years ago, the ability to aggregate, store, retrieve, and present medical information depends greatly on an information infrastructure that accommodates transfer and formatting of structured information. There is currently a great deal of development in key infrastructure components, including storage, enterprise-wide integration, and telecommunication strategies. However, the costs of implementation and support for these new developments are substantial and increasing.

As databases in healthcare increase in number and scope, weaknesses in data collection activities become critical. Lack of uniform definitions, lack of support for data capture at the point of clinical care, struggles related to the coordination of longitudinal follow-up, and issues pertinent to information security and confidentiality require thoughtful evaluation of the constraints of the current practice environment.

The proliferation of information systems has created a situation in which the quantity of data collected strains our ability and resources to analyze and interpret them. As the amount of information steadily increases, it becomes more difficult to select and focus on the data that are truly important for clinical decision-making. It is critical that the questions of focus, function, and form be considered carefully.

Data Quality

The lack of clinical details limits the use of administrative data, in particular, but also can complicate analyses of clinical or research databases. Disease measures may not be captured, illness severity or co-morbidity may be underreported, or definitions may vary by institution or change over time. The development of standards for medical vocabulary and terminology is critical for further progress in the data systems, analysis, and presentation tools. The data collected may also be distorted by payment incentives or other biases. Other problems with data integrity include missing patient data, missing values for certain variables, and incorrect variable values.

The quality of the data is often inversely proportional to the amount of data collected. An important approach to improving data integrity is to specify and enforce a lowest acceptable level of detail. Resources should be focused on collecting the data most useful to clinical and administrative decision-making.

Several techniques of reliability checking can be used to improve the overall quality of data. Consistency and real-life data checks can often be incorporated into the application itself without performance implications. In many cases, it is possible to confirm results by comparing the output with data obtained via another source or a second method. A procedure for auditing a random sample often improves the quality by creating an awareness that data collection is being observed (Hawthorne effect).

Perhaps the most important driver of data quality is the motivation of the individual generating the data. If collecting the data is not an essential part of the actual process of delivery of care, it is usually necessary to provide financial incentives to ensure high-quality and complete data.

Statistical Methods

As interest in monitoring, analyzing, and acting on history has evolved, issues related to statistical methods and clinical decision support systems have become more important. Among the challenges are proper adjustments for differences in baseline characteristics between comparison groups and dealing with missing data. While the comparisons of actual practice with standards of practice have become routine, evaluation of why actual practices and standards of practice differ is considerably more difficult.

The overall objective in both outcomes assessment and process measurement is to derive comparable groups. Comparisons groups are adjusted for factors that lead to treatment selection and factors that lead to outcome of interest, generally by one of two techniques. Stratification permits comparison among patients with similar characteristics. Regression analysis mathematically relates characteristics to develop balanced groups for comparison.

CONCLUSION

There are clear opportunities to improve our ability to extract knowledge from our experiences and to use this knowledge to guide assessments of clinical performance and outcome. Among the opportunities are the better use of real-time tools (including on-line decision support systems), refinement of data collected, and integration of data collected from randomized trials and from administrative and clinical databases.

Clinical information systems should be considered in the context of providing evidence-based medical care. Large databases have the potential to allow individuals and organizations to assimilate and apply all available experience as the basis for healthcare decision-making. However, developing the capacity for evidence-based and cost-effective decision-making depends not only on the database, but also on the skills, culture, and systems within an organization.

Information systems and databases are only pieces of a system whose goals are to use experience to build evidence and to put research into practice. The following scenario is an example of what care be done to improve our ability to deliver better care to patients when an information system is integrated into the process of care.

An important new therapy or treatment strategy is identified based on the results of randomized clinical trial. Clinicians are notified that this therapy is available. Education is provided so that physicians understand which patients are expected to benefit and how the therapy is given, and a consensus is reached that patients who should benefit are to be treated. A plan to implement the therapy is developed. A clinical database is used to identify patients who will benefit. Patients are contacted as needed to ensure eligibility for the new therapy. Arrangements are made to initiate the new therapy in eligible patients. Eligible patients and ongoing treatment are recorded in the database.

There is tremendous potential for the iterative improvement of healthcare. Better application of experience will aid in further refinement of data. This, in turn, will permit the development of enhanced systems and interfaces to provide rapid collection of accurate, complete safety and efficacy data and rapid communication of important results. The ultimate beneficiary will be the patient.

References

1. Pryor DB, Califf RM, Harrell FE Jr, Hlatky MA, Lee KL, Mark DB, Rosati RA: Clinical data bases: Accomplishments and unrealized potential. Med Care 23:623–647, 1985
2. Knoebel SB: Development of a database for clinical use and multicenter collaborative data sharing. J Invas Cardiol 4:99–105, 1992
3. Califf RM. Fortin DF, Tcheng JE, Pryor DB: Goals of clinical databases: Interventional cardiology. In: Roubin G, Philips HR III, O'Neill WW, Califf RM, Stack RS (eds): Interventional Cardiovascular Medicine: Principles and Practice. New York, Churchill Livingstone, 1993
4. Ellerbeck EF, Jencks SF, Radford MJ, Kresowik TF, Craig AS, Gold JA, Krumholz HM, Vogel RE. Quality of care for Medicare patients with acute myocardial infarction: A four-state pilot study from the Cooperative Cardiovascular Project. JAMA 273:1509–1514, 1995
5. Krumholz HM, Radford MJ, Ellerbeck EF, Hennen J, Meehan TP, Petrillo M, Wang Y, Kresowik TF, Jencks SF. Aspirin in the treatment of acute myocardial infarction in elderly Medicare beneficiaries: Patterns of use and outcomes. Circulation 92:2841–2847, 1995

6. Jollis JG, DeLong ER, Peterson ED, Muhlbaier LH, Fortin DF, Califf RM, Mark DB. Outcome of acute myocardial infarction according to the specialty of the admitting physician. N Engl J Med 335:1880–1887, 1996
7. Jollis JG, DeLong ER, Peterson ED, Muhlbaier LH, Fartin DF, Califf RM, Mark DB: Outcome of acute myocardial infarction according to the specialty of the admitting physician. N Engl J Med 335:1880–1887, 1996.
8. Jollis JG, Anstrom KJ, Stafford JA, Mark DB: Mortality following acute myocardial infarction according to physician experience, technical training, and specialty [abstract]. J Am Coll Cardiol 31:363A, 1998
9. Hamm CW, Reimers J, Ischinger T, Rupprecht HJ, Berger J, for the GABI Investigators: A randomized study of coronary angioplasty compared with bypass surgery in patients with symptomatic multivessel coronary disease: German Angioplasty Bypass Surgery Investigation (GABI). N Engl J Med 331:1037–1043, 1994
10. RITA Trial Participants: Coronary angioplasty versus coronary artery bypass surgery: The Randomized Intervention Treatment of Angina (RITA) trial. Lancet 341:573–580, 1993
11. King SB III, Lembo NJ, Weintraub WS, Kosingles AS, Barnhart HX, Kutner MH, Alazraki NP, Guyton RA, Zhao XQ: A randomized trial comparing coronary angioplasty with coronary bypass surgery. N Engl J Med 331:1044–1050, 1994
12. Rodriguez A, Boullon F, Perez-Balino N, Paviotti C, Ligrandi MI, Palacios H: Argentine randomized trial of percutaneous transluminal coronary angioplasty versus coronary artery bypass surgery in multivessel disease (ERACI): In-hospital results and 1-year follow-up. J Am Coll Cardiol 22:1060–1067, 1993
13. CABRI Trial Participants: First-year results of CABRI (Coronary Angioplasty versus Bypass Revascularization Investigation). Lancet 346:1179–1184, 1995
14. The BARI Investigators: Influence of diabetes on 5-year mortality and morbidity in a randomized trial comparing CABG and PTCA in patients with multivessel disease: The Bypass Angioplasty Revascularization Investigation (BARI). Circulation 96:1761–1769, 1997
15. Barsness GW, Peterson ED, Ohman EM, Nelson CL, DeLong ER, Reves SG, Smith PK, Anderson RD, Jones RH, Mark DB, Califf RM: Relationship between diabetes mellitus and long-term survival after coronary bypass and angioplasty. Circulation 96:2551–2556, 1997
16. Detre KM, Rosen AD, Bost JE, Cooger ME, Sutton-Tyrrell K, Holubkhov R, Shamin RS, Frye RL: Contemporary practice of coronary revascularization in U.S. hospitals and hospitals participating in the Bypass Angioplasty Revascularization Investigation (BARI). J Am Coll Cardiol 28:609–615, 1996

Lee A. Fleisher

5 | Principles of Outcome Prediction in Patients with Coronary Artery Disease

The last several years has seen great interest in the concept of evidence-based medicine. In determining the optimal strategy for a given episode of care, physicians frequently use prior knowledge and expert opinion. There is growing concern that much of this knowledge and expert opinion is not rooted in firm scientific proof. The goal of evidence-based medicine is to determine the quality of the scientific proof and to make recommendations based on it. In this chapter, I review some of the general principles of the scientific investigation of risk prediction in cardiovascular disease within this general concept.

For the past 40 years, there has been extensive research into defining those factors that predict future cardiovascular events. Research into the factors that lead to the development of coronary artery disease has been ongoing in large-scale epidemiologic studies. The past several decades has also seen the development of sophisticated tests to detect the extent of coronary artery disease and ventricular function. In particular subsets of patients, specifically those who have sustained a myocardial infarction (MI), sophisticated algorithms have been developed for further risk stratification and intervention.[1] Finally, many interventions based on these risk factors have been evaluated in large-scale randomized clinical trials.

In the area of perioperative cardiovascular outcome research, the development of the science is much less sophisticated. Much of the research is focused on cohort studies to identify those at greatest risk. For noncar-

Outcome Measurements, edited by Kenneth Tuman. Lippincott Williams & Wilkins, Baltimore © 1999

diac surgery, there are no published randomized clinical trials to evaluate the ability of risk prediction to provide information to modify care and improve outcome, although colleagues at Johns Hopkins and I have begun a pilot study, described later in the chapter. The goal of the upcoming decade will be to determine whether further defining predictors of adverse outcomes will result in improved survival. In this chapter, I focus on general principles applied to prediction of cardiovascular outcomes with a specific focus on studies used to define perioperative risk.

DEFINITION OF CARDIOVASCULAR OUTCOMES

Cardiovascular outcomes can generally be divided into 1) the presence of cardiovascular disease and 2) the occurrence of (future) cardiovascular morbidity or mortality. The gold standard for identifying cardiovascular disease is coronary angiography. It is important to remember that coronary angiography is a test of anatomy, not function. Therefore, symptomatology may not directly correlate with the extent of the anatomic stenosis. Many outcome studies have used significant coronary stenosis as the outcome of interest. Yet, from the patient's perspective, morbidity and mortality are the important outcomes.

The definition of a future cardiovascular event differs among the numerous studies because of the variability in the sensitivity and specificity of the diagnostic criteria. Including only irreversible changes in the definition would limit morbidity to a MI and cardiac death. Cardiac death frequently requires confirmation by the presence of myocardial necrosis on autopsy. Death due to arrhythmia is also considered a cardiovascular death, but it may be due to disease other than a significant coronary stenosis. The diagnosis of a MI is even more problematic. The presence of new significant Q waves in two leads of the electrocardiogram (ECG), combined with chest pain and/or an elevation in cardiac isoenzymes, is highly specific for MI. The issue is more difficult for non–Q-wave MI. In the ambulatory setting, the presence of other diagnostic criteria (e.g., chest pain) increases the sensitivity and specificity of cardiac isoenzyme in the diagnosis of a MI. The presence of anginal pain is rare postoperatively because of the masking effects of anesthetics and narcotics. Additionally, the sensitivity and specificity of creatine kinase (CK)-MB for myocardial injury is much lower in surgical patients during the perioperative period than in nonoperative patients. Those patients at greatest risk, i.e., patients undergoing major vascular surgery, can have release of CK-MB from noncardiac sources.[2] Finally, nonspecific ECG changes are common and may not represent true myocardial ischemia.[3] Therefore, the incidence of perioperative MI may vary greatly, in part, because of the different diagnostic criteria employed. Fortunately, recent developments in diagnostic testing for MI have increased the specificity of cardiac isoenzyme tests. Cardiac troponin is now commonly employed in the emergency room setting and is frequently used perioperatively. In the perioperative period, elevated troponin levels may indicate myocardial injury, but the extent of irreversible necrosis is currently not well defined.[4–8] Because of these issues, any study employing MI as an outcome must clearly define the specific diagnostic criteria employed.

Many studies use reversible myocardial events as outcomes of interest. Events such as congestive heart failure and unstable angina are commonly employed in perioperative studies. Again, the definition of unstable angina is unclear because ECG changes are common and pain is rare. Congestive heart failure may occur both from ischemic and nonischemic origins (e.g., fluid overload). Many studies require that congestive heart failure be accompanied by ST-segment changes, but these changes may be either a cause or an effect of the heart failure.

In the absence of a sufficient sample size to detect differences in major morbidity and mortality, some perioperative studies have focused on predicting risk of developing perioperative myocardial ischemia.[9] However, the value of this nonmorbid outcome depends on its relationship with actual morbidity. First, myocardial ischemia has been defined by significant ST-segment changes in these studies. The relationship between ST-segment depression and myocardial ischemia is a function of the prevalence of coronary artery disease in the population. The use of ST-segment monitoring should be considered in the same manner as any noninvasive test; i.e., that a positive result in a low-risk population is most likely a false positive.[10] ST-segment changes in patients at low to moderate risk of coronary artery disease (only one risk factor without known coronary artery disease) are rare and did not correlate with ischemia on a stress test or for subsequent cardiovascular symptoms or events during 2 years of follow-up.[11] Second, not all episodes of myocardial ischemia lead to irreversible myocardial necrosis. Previous studies demonstrating a relationship between duration of ST-segment depression and cardiac morbidity have been interpreted to suggest that prolonged supply-demand mismatches can lead to morbidity.[12,13] An alternative interpretation is that the prolonged ST-segment changes represent an evolving infarction due to an acute coronary thrombosis. This phenomenon is distinct from the other episodes of supply-demand–mediated myocardial ischemia. Therefore, short episodes of ST-segment changes that reflect myocardial ischemia may simply be a normal manifestation of an underlying critical coronary stenosis. In contrast, the event (thrombosis) that leads to myocardial necrosis may be distinct and via a different mechanism. Factors that predict perioperative ST-segment depression may not predict perioperative cardiac morbidity.

TYPES OF STUDIES

Prospective Cohort Studies

There are several study designs, each of which provides different strengths of evidence and degrees of generalizability. Prospective cohort studies involve the identification of a group of subjects who are observed over time for the occurrence of an outcome of interest. The goal is to determine those patients who develop the outcome. If the cohort includes patients free of disease, then those factors that are associated with the development of disease can be discerned. An example of a prospective cohort study related to the development of coronary artery disease is the Framingham Heart Study.[14]

Four decades ago, a cohort of individuals was identified in Framingham, MA.[14] With funding from the National Institutes of Health, these individuals were observed on a predefined schedule to assess baseline medical conditions and physical findings and the subsequent development of coronary artery disease. Numerous risk factors have been found to be associated with a higher incidence of coronary artery disease than those individuals without the risk factors. Examples include hypertension, diabetes, and elevated cholesterol.[15,16]

An example of a prospective cohort study identifying perioperative risk is that of Goldman and colleagues, which led to the development of the Cardiac Risk Index[17] (Table 5–1). Numerous studies have studied large groups of surgical patients above a predefined age and determine those factors that predict risk.[18] Many use multivariate modeling, an analysis technique described later in the chapter, to determine the influence of each of the risk factors to the outcome of interest.

Another example of a prospective cohort study is one in which patients with a known disease are studied for the development of predefined outcomes. Such studies provide the natural history in patients with the disease. An example would be studies of patients who have sustained a MI, in which the value of diagnostic testing for future cardiovascular events can be determined. The studies by Rao et al.[19] and Shah et al.[20], which evaluated the incidence of perioperative reinfarction in patients who had previously sustained a MI, are examples of this study design.

Although prospective cohort studies have important value in identifying risk factors for the outcome of interest, there are significant limitations. The selection of the cohort of interest can significantly affect the results obtained. The larger the cohort, the more generalizable the results. A second bias is that many patients may be lost to follow-up. In perioperative studies, this may not be an important issue for short-term outcomes, but it may become important in long-term (survival) outcomes. Follow-up is always an issue in large-scale epidemiological

TABLE 5–1. COMPUTATION OF THE CARDIAC RISK INDEX

Criteria	Multivariate Discriminant Function Coefficient	Points
History		
Age >70 yr	0.191	5
MI in previous 6 mo	0.384	10
Physical examination		
S_3 gallop or JVD	0.451	11
Important VAS	0.119	3
Electrocardiogram		
Rhythm other than sinus or PACs on last preoperative ECG	0.283	7
>5 PVCs/min documented at any time before operation	0.278	7
General status		
PO_2 <60 or PCO_2 >50 mm Hg, K <3.0 or HCO_3^- <2 mEq/L BUN >50 or Cr >3.0 mg/dL, abnormal SGOT, signs of chronic liver disease, or patient bedridden from noncardiac causes	0.132	3
Operation		
Intraperitoneal, intrathoracic, or aortic operation	0.123	3
Emergency operation	0.167	4
Total possible		53

MI, myocardial infarction; JVD, jugular-vein distention; VAS, valvular aortic stenosis; PACs, premature atrial contractions; ECG, electrocardiogram; BUN, blood urea nitrogen; Cr, creatinine; SGOT, serum glutamic oxalacetic transaminase.
From Goldman et al.[17] with permission.

studies of the development of coronary artery disease. Finally, the importance of a risk factor depends on the completeness of the data. For example, if the presence of severe angina was not included in the database, then it could not be a risk factor, and other factors may appear to be more important.

Randomized Clinical Trial

A specific example of a prospective cohort study is the randomized clinical trial. Randomized clinical trials represent the gold standard for evidence of causation. They have defined inclusion and exclusion criteria, treatment protocols, and outcomes of interest. They are usually either single- or double-blinded (both patient and physician) and are designed to test the effect of a new drug or intervention. They rarely are used as a means of identifying risk, but they may be used to determine whether that risk factor is truly linked via a causal relationship or simply an association. For example, high cholesterol levels are associated with an increased incidence of the development of coronary artery disease in multiple epidemiological and prospective cohort series. With the advent of the statin class of drugs, the effect of lowering cholesterol levels on the progression or development of coronary disease can be established.[21] Because such trials have shown a beneficial effect, the evidence supporting the link between elevated cholesterol levels and coronary disease is firmly established. In the perioperative period, hypothermia has been associated with an increased incidence of perioperative ischemia, a surrogate marker for morbidity.[22] In a subsequent randomized clinical trial, the use of forced-air warming to maintain normothermia was associated with a significantly lower incidence of perioperative morbid cardiac events.[23] Therefore, randomized clinical trials are frequently performed after the results of a prospective cohort study to confirm the findings of an association.

Randomized clinical trials derive their strength from an evidence-based perspective because of their high degree of internal validity: i.e., the randomization scheme and use of placebo (or accepted alternative treatments) provide strong evidence that the results are related to the intervention. Importantly, these trials have a lower degree of external validity because the intervention may not behave in the same manner when it is diffused into a more heterogeneous population in which treatment is not defined by protocol. This differentiation distinguishes the intervention's efficacy under strict protocols versus effectiveness under real-world conditions. It has also led to large-scale clinical effectiveness trials in which care is much less protocolized. A more complete discussion of the strengths and weaknesses of randomized trials versus cohort studies of interventions can be found in Chapter 2.

Case-Controlled Studies

Retrospective studies involve identifying patients who have sustained an outcome and then defining risk factors associated with the outcome. An example of a retrospective design is a case-control study. Case-control studies identify patients with the outcome of interest. Frequently, these patients may be included as part of a prospective cohort study. The prevalence of a risk factor in the patients with the outcome (case) is then compared with the prevalence of the risk factor in matched controls, so that the efficiency and power of the results can be maximized. The ratio of cases to controls can be varied, with greater power with an increasing number of controls.

Case-controlled studies are extremely useful as a means of reducing potential bias as a cause of the association between a risk factor and outcome. It is the method by which the increased cardiovascular risk associated with homocysteine was initially noted. It can also be used to evaluate interventions for which a randomized clinical trial would be unethical or impossible to undertake. A recent example would be the risk associated with a pulmonary artery catheter. As part of a prospective evaluation of end-of-life decisions (SUPPORT Trial[23a]), patients with a pulmonary artery catheter were compared with patients who did not receive a pulmonary artery catheter matched on multiple factors after completion of the trial. The investigators performed this analysis because no prospective trial could be performed because of clinician bias, which led to their refusal to allow their patients to undergo randomization. Based on the analysis of the SUPPORT Trial data, the investigators reported a higher mortality rate in those patients who received a pulmonary catheter than in the matched controls. Rather than providing definitive evidence of causation, the Trial supports the ethics of performing a prospective randomized trial of the pulmonary artery catheter.

Case-control studies are subject to a number of biases. The exact definitions of cases and controls can influence the analysis. Frequently, patients are matched on age and gender, but other factors may play an important role. It is also critical that the exposure or intervention precedes the outcome and that a dose-response gradient further confirms the relationship.

Use of Administrative Databases

When extremely large sample sizes are needed, administrative databases may be among the most cost-effective approaches. Examples of administrative databases include Medicare claims files, private insurance company claims, and hospital electronic records. These databases include a small number of data points on an extremely large number of subjects. For example, the Medicare database includes both financial data and International Classification of Diseases-9 (ICD-9; disease) and Current Procedural Terminology (procedure) codes for each patient. They also include information regarding location of care and provider type.

Administrative databases have been used extensively in the area of utilization of cardiovascular resources in relation to outcome. The idea of assessing appropriateness of care has been studied since the original report by Wennberg and Gittelsohn[24] assessing different rates of tonsillectomy utilization in New England. Investigators have been very interested in assessing the use of both coronary angiography and coronary revascularization in different regions of the United States and in different countries.[25,26] These databases also contain mortality data for comparison. Using such methodology, investigators have suggested that the increased use of cardiovascular resources in the United States is not associated with improved outcome when compared with Canada.[27] The Medicare claims files are now being used extensively to benchmark rates of mortality and major complications after coronary bypass surgery. Hospitals can compare their rates with those of neighboring and competing hospitals. Information regarding length of stay and cost is also available. National standards have been set by many of the actuarial companies using these data.

The Medicare claims data have also been used for assessing risk after vascular surgery. Mortality after vascular surgery varies by both hospital and surgeon, as demonstrated by such analyses. Fleisher and colleagues[11] have investigated the value of preoperative testing before major vascular surgery. By having access to Medicare claims files in which 1-year follow-up is available, the incidence of 30-day and 1-year mortality after major vascular surgery could be evaluated based on the preoperative use of diagnostic testing and coronary interventions. The advantage of such an analysis is that it includes a cross-section of hospitals. Therefore, the significant publication bias of reports from academic medical centers is minimized.

Although there are many benefits to the analysis of administrative databases, there are also significant shortcomings. Potential selection bias is difficult or impossible to determine. There is also difficulty in risk adjustment, which could account for much of the variability in outcome. Attempts have been made to develop risk-adjustment measures; one example is the Charlson Index of Comorbidities.[28] Charlson and colleagues[28] developed a scale for predicting mortality from breast cancer based on the presence of comorbidities within the previous 1 year. By analyzing ICD-9 codes related to comorbidities for a 1-year period or those present during a single episode of care for a given individual, an index can be defined. The rate of mortality or major morbidity can then be adjusted to account for these factors.

Another major limitation of administrative databases is the reliance on correct coding. As most clinicians are aware, discharge coding is frequently incorrect. Some investigators review actual patient's charts to confirm the accuracy of the data, but this is rarely an available solution. Therefore, there may be bias in those data. There also may be problems in the assessments of outcomes. Mortality is a hard outcome, but even mortality data may be problematic. For example, out-of-hospital mortality is not reported in the Medicare data set. Investigators would be required to cross-reference patients with the national death registry. Nonfatal outcomes are even more problematic. A recent analysis of perioperative MI rates after vascular surgery showed the incidence to be 25%

of the reported mortality. Because this is incongruent with known data from clinical trials, it most likely reflects the omission of this diagnostic code from the discharge summary. Frequently, comorbidities are also not included in the discharge summary, which makes analysis of a comorbidity index much more difficult. In conclusion, administrative databases provide important tools for investigators to study practice patterns and mortality rates for cardiovascular services in large cohorts of unselected patients, but the data contain biases related to the method of collection. Most investigators believe that such analyses generate hypothesis rather than provide definitive evidence or conclusions.

TESTING TO DETERMINE THE PRESENCE OF CORONARY ARTERY DISEASE OR FUTURE CARDIAC MORBIDITY

In patients with risk factors or symptoms, further evaluation may be required to confirm the presence of coronary artery disease. In interpreting the results of any test, it is important to understand the properties of the test. For coronary artery disease, the gold standard is coronary angiography. Importantly, angiography quantitates the static anatomic lesions. Both symptoms and signs of myocardial ischemia do not necessarily correlate with the extent of a coronary stenosis.

In interpreting studies related to diagnostic testing, it is important to understand the differences among sensitivity, specificity, positive predictive value, and negative predictive value (Table 5–2). Within this context, it is important to define the outcome of interest. For the presence and extent of coronary artery disease, noninvasive tests are compared with the coronary angiogram. In the case of risk prediction, the outcome of interest is frequently sustaining a future cardiovascular event, not the presence of disease. Further complicating the matter is the variability in the definition of a cardiovascular event as described above. Although sensitivity and specificity can be calculated for a future event, the predictive value of the test is the characteristic most frequently reported.

Within the context of this argument, it is important to know that the sensitivity and specificity of a diagnostic test are specific attributes of the test. In contrast, the predictive value of the test is a function of the probability of the important outcome or disease in the population studied. The probability that the disease exists in patients with a positive or negative test is a function of the probability of disease or event in the population and the sensitivity and specificity of the diagnostic test. This concept is termed Bayes' theorem.[10] It is especially relevant in predicting future cardiovascular events. In this case, the predictive value of the test is a function of the overall probability of the event for that population.

Table 5-2. Definitions Commonly Used Terms in Epidemiology and Decision-Making

Test Result	Disease State	
	Present	Absent
Positive	a (true positive)	b (false positive)
Negative	c (false negative)	d (true negative)
Prevalence (prior probability)	(a + c)/(a + b + c + d)	All patients with the disease/all patients tested
Sensitivity (true-positive rate)	a/(a + c)	True-positive test results/all patients with the disease
Specificity (true-negative rate)	d/(b + d)	True-negative test results/all patients without the disease
False-negative rate	c/(a + c)	False-negative test results/all patients with the disease
False-positive rate	b/(b + d)	False-positive test results/all patients without the disease
Positive predictive value	a/(a + b)	True-positive test results/all positive test results
Negative predictive value	d/(c + d)	True-negative test results/all patients with negative results
Overall accuracy	(a + d)/(a + b + c + d)	True-positive + true-negative test results/all tests
Likelihood ratio for a positive test	$\dfrac{a/(a+c)}{b/(b+d)}$	True-positive rate/false-positive rate
Likelihood ratio for a negative test	$\dfrac{d/(b+d)}{c/(a+c)}$	True-negative rate/false-negative rate

Adapted from Fauci AS, Braunwals E, Isselbacher KJ, et al. (eds.): Harrison's Principles of Internal Medicine 14th ed, p. 10, McGraw-Hill, 1998.

In terms of Bayes' theorem, a noninvasive test is most useful in patients at moderate risk. This is because no noninvasive test is 100% sensitive or specific. If the population of interest has a low probability of coronary disease, then the test has minimal discriminatory ability. In such a scenario, a positive test is most likely a false positive. If the population of interest has a high probability of coronary artery disease, then a negative test is most likely a false negative. The test only provides significant predictive value in the population at moderate risk of disease (Figure 5–1). This was first shown by Eagle and colleagues.[29] Two hundred consecutive patients undergoing vascular surgery were studied, and five clinical risk factors were identified (Q waves on ECG, angina, diabetes mellitus, age >70 years, and active treatment for ventricular ectopic activity) (Figure 5–2). Patients without clinical risk factors had only a 3% incidence of perioperative morbidity, and noninvasive testing could not further stratify risk. Similarly, patients with three or more clinical risk factors had a 50% morbidity, and noninvasive testing could not further stratify risk. Preoperative dipyridamole thallium imaging was, however, useful in the group at moderate risk (one or two risk factors). This study helps to explain differences in predictive values reported between consecutive and selective patient series.

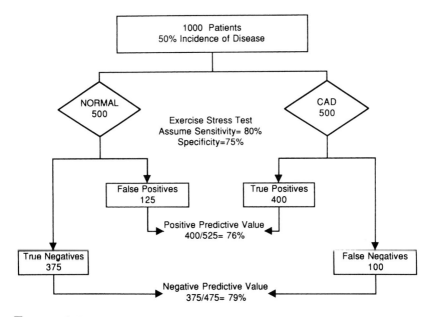

FIGURE 5–1. A representative exercise stress test evaluated in a population with a 50% incidence of disease. In such a population at moderate risk, the positive and negative predictive values are high (76% and 79%, respectively). CAD, coronary artery disease.

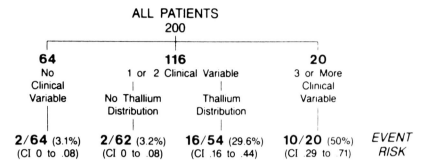

FIGURE 5–2. The value of preoperative testing in a cohort of 200 patients undergoing major vascular surgery. Five clinical variables were identified (angina, ventricular ectopic activity, diabetes, Q waves, and age >70 years). Only in those patients with one or two clinical variables (moderate risk) was noninvasive testing of value in further defining risk. Reproduced with permission from Reference 29.

The use of a Bayesian model to evaluate the role of preoperative testing was shown by L'Italien and colleagues.[30] Using data collected from more than 1000 patients who had undergone preoperative dipyridamole thallium imaging, the pretest (baseline) probability of an event could be calculated in a manner similar to cardiac risk indices, whereby clinical risk factors each are associated with a certain numerical weight, which can be added to determine overall risk. The results of dipyridamole thallium imaging could then be used to modify the risk and to determine the posttest probability of an event. In this manner, clinical risk factors can be used to determine whether the test will change the probability of morbidity, and the value of a Bayesian approach to testing can best be illustrated.

DATA ANALYSIS

The method of analysis of the data using statistical tests can have a significant impact on the interpretation of the results. It is important to use the appropriate statistical tests for any given data set (in-depth discussion of this is beyond the scope of this chapter). An overview of how to choose a statistical test is shown in Table 5–3. Most of these tests are now available in commercial packages for a personal computer.

The definition of statistical significance traditionally refers to a P value <0.05. This value denotes that the probability of finding a similar difference between two treatments or a significant association with an outcome occurs by chance in less than 1 in 20 instances. Although this statistical relationship may exist, it is important to determine whether a clinical relationship exists. If such a relationship is improbable, it is im-

TABLE 5-3. OVERVIEW OF HOW TO CHOOSE STATISTICAL TESTS

Type of Measure	Comparison of Two Groups of Different Individuals with Each Other	Comparison of Same Individuals with Themselves—Two Measurements on Each	Comparison of Three or More Groups of Different Individuals	Comparison of Same Individuals with Themselves—Three of More Measurements on Each	Association of Two Different Variables with Each Other—Each Measured in the Same Individual
Continuous and either normally distributed or measured in many subjects (e.g., blood pressure)	Unpaired t-test	Paired t-test	Analysis of variance	Repeated measures analysis of variance	Pearson correlation coefficient or linear regression
Ordered but in a few subjects or not normally distributed	Mann-Whitney rank sum test	Wilcoxon signed-rank test	Kruskal-Wallis statistic	Friedman statistic	Spearman rank correlation coefficient
Categorical—often dichotomous (two categories) and usually five or fewer categories	χ^2 test or Fisher's exact test	McNemar's test	χ^2 test	Cochrane Q	Contingency

Adapted with permission from Glantz, SA: Primer of Biostatics. 3rd ed. McGraw-Hill, 1992.

portant to further validate the results. If the results are not statistically significant, then a type II (β) error may exist. A β error occurs because the study was of insufficient size to detect a statistical relationship.

One particular type of statistical analysis frequently performed in studies of risk prediction is the multivariate analysis. Multivariate analysis is useful in determining the importance of independent factors for an outcome. It allows the investigator to adjust for potentially confounding factors. If the outcome is continuous (e.g., days in the intensive care unit) and the predictive variables are also continuous (e.g., blood pressure) then linear regression techniques are used. If the outcome variable is dichotomous (e.g., life or death) then logistic regression techniques are most useful. Examples of multivariate analysis include the Goldman Cardiac Risk Index and many cardiac surgery risk indices. If the outcome is in more than two ordered categories (e.g., no complications, MI, death), then discriminative analysis is performed. The basic method is to create an equation that weights the various predictive factors and adds them to provide a score. Factors are included or eliminated from the model based on statistical and biological significance. With many of the commercial software packages, there is a stepwise process of either adding or subtracting each factor and evaluating the statistical significance of the overall model.

Although multivariate analysis is a very powerful technique in the area of risk prediction, there are several potential confounders, as described throughout this chapter. It is important to have a complete list of potential risk factors for a given outcome because some critical factors may be overlooked. Additionally, if the risk factors are present in a low incidence in the population studied, then such risk factors may not achieve statistical significance. For example, Canadian Cardiovascular Association Class IV angina was not a significant risk factor in the Goldman Cardiac Risk Index. At the time of the study, few such patients underwent surgery and therefore were not present in sufficient quantities in the analysis. This illustrates the importance of including biological significance in the decision to incorporate or eliminate a factor from the model. The number of patients with an adverse event affects the number of risk factors that achieve statistical significance in the model. Therefore, large samples with more adverse events will allow more robust modeling. Studies in which only a few adverse events occur have a limited ability to determine predictors of adverse outcome.

Meta-Analysis

Traditionally, authors have reviewed the literature in a nonsystematic manner and written chapters or articles incorporating their own opinions regarding risk prediction or the value of an intervention. A more formal process might include the use of a consensus conference, but this does not represent a truly evidence-based perspective of practice. More recently, practice guidelines and evidence-based articles attempt to review the literature in a systematic fashion. As part of the selection criteria for the literature, the investigator defines the methods of the literature search (MEDLINE search words, years included, secondary search of references from articles identified). Criteria for the inclusion of articles are established *a priori*. Articles are prepared that outline the strength of evidence to support various conclusions based on this formal review.

When multiple studies are performed to evaluate a given technology or intervention, a more formal synthesis can be produced under the heading of meta-analysis. Meta-analysis has been defined as a quantitative summary of research in a particular area and the practice of using statistical methods to combine the outcome of a series of different experiments or investigations. Classic meta-analysis includes randomized clinical trials. There is currently a debate in the literature regarding the appropriateness of including nonrandomized or cohort trials.[31] In the area of risk prediction, most of the literature represents such cohort trials. Two meta-analyses have been published regarding the value of preoperative testing for noncardiac surgery.[32,33] Both demonstrated the positive predictive value of the diagnostic test, with the highest predictive value being afforded to dobutamine stress testing, but including significant overlap with dipyridamole thallium imaging. The potential value of meta-analytic techniques is best illustrated with regard to the use of streptokinase for acute MI.[34] Several small trials demonstrating the efficacy of streptokinase in improving outcome after MI had initially been performed. If a cumulative meta-analysis was performed after the smaller trials, a clear and significant benefit could be demonstrated. However, review of textbooks of cardiology from the same period does not demonstrate that streptokinase was recommended. It took several more years and large-scale trials before streptokinase became a routine recommendation (Figure 5–3). Therefore, performance of a meta-analysis would have resulted in an early recommendation for this potentially life-saving therapy.

SPECIFIC ISSUES RELATED TO THE PERIOPERATIVE PERIOD

Because virtually all of the studies related to predicting outcome in the perioperative period employ analysis of a cohort of patients, there are certain basic principles that affect the generalizability and limitations of the findings. Most importantly, virtually all studies begin with a

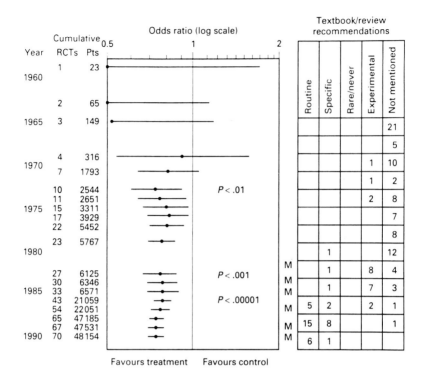

FIGURE 5–3. The effect of additional randomized clinical trials on a cumulative meta-analysis of the beneficial effects of thrombolytic therapy after an acute myocardial infarction. If the point estimate and confidence interval lie entirely to the left of 1.0, then there is a significant benefit to the intervention. The table to the right lists the number of recommendations in textbooks to utilize thrombolytic therapy. There is a long delay between the routine recommendation of its use and the point at which a meta-analysis would have demonstrated a statistically significant benefit. Reproduced with permission from Antman EM, Lau J, Kupelnick B, Mosteller F, Chalmers TC: A comparison of results of meta-analyses of randomized control trials and recommendations of clinical experts: Treatments for myocardial infarction. JAMA 268:240–248, 1992.

selection bias. This may include either a referral bias to the hospital or referral bias for the study. None of the published studies related to preoperative evaluation evaluate a geographic cohort, but rather a hospital cohort. Particularly in the United States, referral patterns may be based on the expertise of the setting, in addition to geographic issues. For example, the patients at highest risk may be sent to university hospitals, whereas patients at lower risk may be seen in community-based settings. In addition to selective admission of patients to a particular hospital or surgeon, there maybe a referral bias with respect to entry into the study. Many studies evaluate consecutive patients who were referred to a preoperative screening clinic. An alternative approach has been to enroll patients referred for preoperative diagnostic testing. There are both positive and negative aspects of studying referred patients with regard to diagnostic testing. Two recent studies illustrate the reduced value of noninvasive testing when consecutive surgical patients are studied, as opposed to restricting the evaluation to those at moderate risk. Mangano and colleagues[35] studied 60 consecutive patients undergoing vascular surgery and reported a positive predictive value of 27% for adverse cardiac events, a negative predictive value of 82%, and no net discriminative ability of the test. Baron and colleagues[36] studied the largest (457) consecutive population of patients undergoing abdominal aortic surgery and were also unable to demonstrate an association between thallium redistribution and perioperative cardiac morbidity. Both studies illustrate the low positive predictive value and significant incidence of morbidity in patients with negative test results when consecutive patients are studied. In contrast, Vanzetto et al.[37] observed a cohort of consecutive abdominal aortic surgery patients and performed dipyridamole thallium imaging only in the subset of patients with more than one clinical or ECG cardiac risk variables. The results of the test were not made available to the clinicians. Major cardiac events occurred in 23% of patients with a reversible thallium defect and in 1% of patients without reversible thallium defects in clinically high-cardiac risk patients, demonstrating significant prognostic value for cardiac events over that provided by clinical variables alone. Therefore, preoperative testing continues to be widely applied to stratify perioperative risk if used appropriately.

    An additional issue regarding cohort studies revolves around the concept of the intraoperative period as a "black box." Many of these studies make the assumption that care cannot be modified based on preoperative information. Such an assumption is counter to the basic premise of the preoperative evaluation: information from the evaluation will be used to modify care and improve outcome. Therefore, those factors that are initially identified as placing the patient at greatest risk may no longer be shown to be significant on subsequent evaluation. Additionally, if the information is available to the clinician and care is modified, then the factor may not be significantly associated with poor outcome. If the factor is subsequently ignored or unknown (as may be the case if preoperative cardiovascular testing is eliminated), then the frequency of perioperative events may increase.

    Many investigators have argued that the value of preoperative noninvasive cardiovascular testing before noncardiac surgery cannot be firmly established because of the lack of randomized controlled trials. Specifically, it is unknown whether further defining the extent of risk will affect perioperative and long-term outcome. In an attempt to investigate the importance of preoperative testing, I and colleagues at

Johns Hopkins Bayview Medical Center have undertaken a randomized trial in which patients either undergo testing per the American Heart Association/American College of Cardiology testing guidelines or undergo major vascular surgery without further evaluation. Hopefully, the results of such a study will further define the value of preoperative risk stratification.

DECISION ANALYSIS

In the absence of randomized clinical trials to assess the value of preoperative risk stratification, decision analysis offers an alternative method. Decision analysis is an explicit analytic tool designed to facilitate complex clinical therapeutic or diagnostic decisions in which many variables must be considered simultaneously.[38–40] The steps in decision analysis begin with constructing a decision tree. A decision tree is a map of all relevant courses of action and their associated outcomes. The tree is built from left to right and consists of nodes, branches, and outcomes. A decision node is a branch point representing a diagnostic or therapeutic decision, which is conventionally depicted as a square. A branch point of a chance outcome not directly controlled by the physician is conventionally represented as a circle. Outcomes are depicted as rectangles or triangles.

Two decision analyses on the value of preoperative cardiovascular testing before major vascular surgery have been published (Figure 5–4).

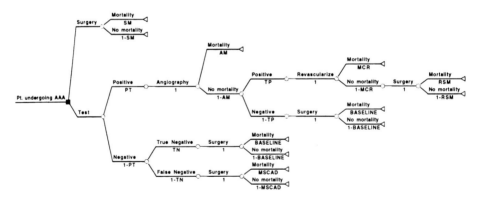

FIGURE 5–4. A representative decision algorithm evaluating the decision between vascular surgery alone or coronary artery revascularization before vascular surgery. There are currently no randomized trials to address the optimal strategy. By outlining the multiple decision points at which a patient can sustain mortality by choosing to undergo coronary revascularization first, the optimal strategy for preoperative evaluation can be demonstrated. Specifically, variation in mortalities at each decision point can change the optimal strategy. Reproduced with permission from Reference 41.

Both assumed that patients with significant coronary artery disease would undergo coronary artery bypass grafting before noncardiac surgery. Both models found that the optimal decision was sensitive to local morbidity and mortality rates within the clinically observed range (Figure 5–5). These models suggest that preoperative testing for the purpose of coronary revascularization is not the optimal strategy if perioperative morbidity and mortality are low.

The primary cost (both in dollars and morbidity) of preoperative testing and revascularization is the revascularization procedure itself. Therefore, the indications for revascularization and, thus, the frequency of its use, has a significant impact on the model. Potential long-term benefits of coronary revascularization in this population were not included in the analysis, potentially causing bias against the revascularization arm. If long-term survival is included in the models, then coro-

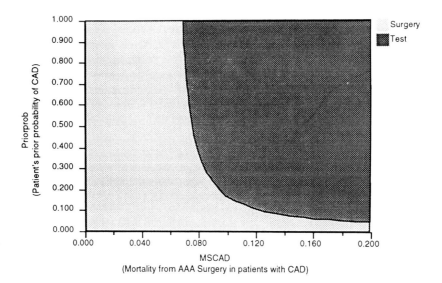

FIGURE 5–5. An example of a two-way sensitivity analysis based on the decision analysis proposed in Figure 4 demonstrating the optimal preoperative strategy of surgery alone or coronary revascularization before vascular surgery. Two of the critical variables in the decision analysis are varied within the clinically relevant range. As the probability of mortality from coronary revascularization increases, then vascular surgery alone becomes the preferred strategy. In contrast, as the probability of mortality from aortic surgery in patients with significant coronary artery disease increases, then coronary revascularization before vascular surgery becomes the optimal strategy. The average mortality for vascular surgery in patients with significant coronary artery disease is 9.5%, which suggests that the strategy with the lowest mortality is very sensitive to local morbidity and mortality. However, if long-term mortality is included in the model, the coronary revascularization may prove to be more beneficial. Reproduced with permission from Reference 41.

nary revascularization may lead to improved overall outcome and be a cost-effective intervention. The strength of decision analysis is that numerous inputs can be included in the model. For example, 80-year-old diabetic patients with significant comorbid diseases may gain few additional life years and may actually experience a decrease in the quality of their final years by undergoing coronary revascularization. In contrast, 55-year-old patients with an abdominal aortic aneurysm who are found to have occult left main disease would have a substantial increase in both the length and quality of their life from preoperative cardiovascular testing and coronary revascularization. Therefore, identification of appropriate patients with multivessel disease or a significant left main coronary artery stenosis amenable to surgery with an acceptable risk should prompt coronary artery bypass grafting before noncardiac surgery. In this instance, the coronary revascularization procedure is justified based on long-term benefit, and performing it before noncardiac surgery reduces the risk of a fatal or nonfatal perioperative MI.

SUMMARY

The science of risk assessment has now focused on an evidence-based approach. In the population of nonsurgical patients, prospective cohort trials have identified a number of important risk factors. Trials of therapeutic interventions are now ongoing to test the ability to modify this risk. The science is less well developed in the area of preoperative risk stratification and relies primarily on cohort trials using multivariate analysis. In the absence of randomized trials, decision analysis has been employed to determine whether risk stratification and potential interventions will lead to improved outcomes.

References

1. Ryan TJ, Anderson JL, Antman EM, Braniff BA, Brooks NH, Califf RM, Hillis LD, Hiratzka LF, Rapaport E, Riegel BJ, Russell RO, Smith EE III, Weaver WD: ACC/AHA guidelines for the management of patients with acute myocardial infarction: Executive summary—A report of the American College of Cardiology/American Heart Association Task Force on Practice Guidelines (Committee on Management of Acute Myocardial Infarction). Circulation 94: 2341–2350, 1996
2. Mangano DT: Beyond CK-MB: Biochemical markers for perioperative myocardial infarction. Anesthesiology 81:1317–1320, 1994

3. Breslow MJ, Miller CF, Parker SD, Walman AT, Rogers MC: Changes in T-wave morphology following anesthesia and surgery: A common recovery-room phenomenon. Anesthesiology 64:398–402, 1986
4. Metzler H, Gries M, Rehak P, Lang T, Fruhwald S, Toller W: Perioperative myocardial cell injury: the role of troponins. Br J Anaesth 78:386–390, 1997
5. Lopez-Jimenez F, Goldman L, Sacks DB, Thomas EJ, Johnson PA, Cook EF, Lee TH: Prognostic value of cardiac troponin T after non-cardiac surgery: 6-month follow-up data. J Am Coll Cardiol 29: 1241–1245, 1997
6. Hake U, Schmid FX, Iversen S, Dahm M, Mayer E, Hafner G, Oelert H: Troponin T: A reliable marker of perioperative myocardial infarction? Eur J Cardiothorac Surg 7:628–633, 1993
7. Lee TH, Thomas EJ, Ludwig LE, Sacks DB, Johnson PA, Donaldson MC, Cook EF, Pedan A, Kuntz KM, Goldman L: Troponin T as a marker for myocardial ischemia in patients undergoing major noncardiac surgery. Am J Cardiol 77:1031–1036, 1996
8. Adams J, Sicard GA, Allen BT, Bridwell KH, Lenke LG, Davila-Roman VG, Bodor GS, Ladenson JH, Jaffe AS: Diagnosis of perioperative myocardial infarction with measurement of cardiac troponin I . N Engl J Med 330:670–674, 1994
9. Hollenberg M, Mangano DT, Browner WS, London MJ, Tubau JF, Tateo IM: Predictors of postoperative myocardial ischemia in patients undergoing noncardiac surgery: The Study of Perioperative Ischemia Research. JAMA 268:205–209, 1992
10. Shuman P: Bayes' theorem: A review. Cardiol Clin 2:319–328, 1984
11. Fleisher LA, Eagle KA, Shaffer T, Anderson G: Mortality after major vascular surgery: Analysis of the Medicare database [abstract]. Anesth Analg 84(Suppl):43, 1997
12. Landesberg G, Luria MH, Cotev S, Eidelman LA, Anner H, Mosseri M, Schechter D, Assaf J, Erel J, Berlatzky Y: Importance of long-duration postoperative ST-segment depression in cardiac morbidity after vascular surgery. Lancet 341:715–719, 1993
13. Fleisher LA, Nelson AH, Rosenbaum SH: Postoperative myocardial ischemia: Etiology of cardiac morbidity or manifestation of underlying disease. J Clin Anesth 7:97–102, 1995
14. Lerner D, Kannel W: Patterns of coronary heart disease morbidity and mortality in the sexes: A 26-year follow-up of the Framingham population. Am Heart J 113:383–390, 1986
15. Kannel W, Abbott R: Incidence and prognosis of unrecognized myocardial infarction: An update on the Framingham Study. N Engl J Med 311:1144–1147, 1984
16. Castelli W, Anderson K: A population at risk: Prevalence of high

cholesterol levels in hypertensive patients in the Framingham study. Am J Med 80(Suppl 2A):23, 1986
17. Goldman L, Caldera DL, Nussbaum SR, Southwick FS, Krogstad D, Murray B, Burke DS, O'Malley TA, Goroll AH, Caplan CH, Nolan J, Carabello B, Slater EE: Multifactorial index of cardiac risk in noncardiac surgical procedures. N Engl J Med 297:845–850, 1977
18. Shah KB, Kleinman BS, Rao T, Jacobs HK, Mestan K, Schaafsma M: Angina and other risk factors in patients with cardiac diseases undergoing noncardiac operations. Anesth Analg 70:240–247, 1990
19. Rao TLK, Jacobs KH, El-Etr AA: Reinfarction following anesthesia in patients with myocardial infarction. Anesthesiology 59:499–505, 1983
20. Shah KB, Kleinman BS, Sami H, Patel I, Rao T: Reevaluation of perioperative myocardial infarction in patients with prior myocardial infarction undergoing noncardiac operations. Anesth Analg 71:231–235, 1990
21. Simes RJ: Prospective meta-analysis of cholesterol-lowering studies: The Prospective Pravastatin Pooling (PPP) Project and the Cholesterol Treatment Trialists (CTT) Collaboration. Am J Cardiol 76:122C–126C, 1995
22. Frank SM, Beattie C, Christopherson R, Norris EJ, Perler BA, Williams GM, Gottlieb SO: Unintentional hypothermia is associated with postoperative myocardial ischemia: The Perioperative Ischemia Randomized Anesthesia Trial Study Group. Anesthesiology 78:468–476, 1993
23. Frank SM, Fleisher LA, Breslow MJ, Higgins MS, Olson KF, Kelly S, Beattie C: Perioperative maintenance of normothermia reduces the incidence of morbid cardiac events: A randomized clinical trial. JAMA 277:1127–1134, 1997
23a. Connors AF Jr, Speroff T, Dawson NV, et al: The effectiveness of right heart catheterization in the initial care of critically ill patients. SUPPORT Investigators. JAMA 276:889–897, 1996
24. Wennberg JE, Gittelsohn A: Health care delivery in Maine. I. Patterns of use of common surgical procedures. J Maine Med Assoc 66:123–130,149, 1975
25. Jollis JG, Peterson ED, DeLong ER, Mark DB, Collins SR, Muhlbaier LH, Pryor DB: The relation between the volume of coronary angioplasty procedures at hospitals treating Medicare beneficiaries and short-term mortality. N Engl J Med 331:1625–1629, 1994
26. Guadagnoli E, Hauptman PJ, Ayanian JZ, Pashos CL, McNeil BJ, Cleary PD: Variation in the use of cardiac procedures after acute myocardial infarction. N Engl J Med 333:573–578, 1995
27. Tu JV, Pashos CL, Naylor CD, Chen E, Normand SL, Newhouse JP, McNeil BJ: Use of cardiac procedures and outcomes in elderly

patients with myocardial infarction in the United States and Canada. N Engl J Med 336:1500–1505, 1997
28. Charlson ME, Pompei P, Ales KL, MacKenzie CR: A new method of classifying prognostic comorbidity in longitudinal studies: Development and validation. J Chronic Dis 40:373–383, 1987
29. Eagle KA, Coley CM, Newell JB, Brewster DC, Darling RC, Strauss HW, Guiney TE, Boucher CA: Combining clinical and thallium data optimizes preoperative assessment of cardiac risk before major vascular surgery. Ann Intern Med 110:859–866, 1989
30. L'Italien GJ, Paul SD, Hendel RC, Leppo JA, Cohen MC, Fleisher LA, Brown KA, Zarich SW, Cambria RP, Cutler BS, Eagle KA: Development and validation of a Bayesian model for perioperative cardiac risk assessment in a cohort of 1,081 vascular surgical candidates. J Am Coll Cardiol 27:779–786, 1996
31. Shapiro S: Meta-analysis/Shmeta-analysis. Am J Epidemiol 140:771–778, 1994
32. Mantha S, Roizen MF, Barnard J, Thisted RA, Ellis JE, Foss J: Relative effectiveness of four preoperative tests for predicting adverse cardiac outcomes after vascular surgery: A meta-analysis. Anesth Analg 79:422–433, 1994
33. Shaw LJ, Eagle KA, Gersh BJ, Miller DD: Meta-analysis of intravenous dipyridamole-thallium-201 imaging (1985 to 1994) and dobutamine echocardiography (1991 to 1994) for risk stratification before vascular surgery. J Am Coll Cardiol 27:787–798, 1996
34. Antman EM, Lau J, Kupelnick B, Mosteller F, Chalmers TC: A comparison of results of meta-analyses of randomized control trials and recommendations of clinical experts: Treatments for myocardial infarction. JAMA 268:240–248, 1992
35. Mangano DT, London MJ, Tubau JF, Browner WS, Hollenberg M, Krupski W, Layug EL, Massie B: Dipyridamole thallium-201 scintigraphy as a preoperative screening test: A reexamination of its predictive potential—Study of Perioperative Ischemia Research Group. Circulation 84:493–502, 1991
36. Baron JF, Mundler O, Bertrand M, Vicaut E, Barre E, Godet G, Samama CM, Coriat P, Kieffer E, Viars P: Dipyridamole-thallium scintigraphy and gated radionuclide angiography to assess cardiac risk before abdominal aortic surgery. N Engl J Med 330:663–669, 1994
37. Vanzetto G, Machecourt J, Blendea D, Fagret D, Borrel E, Magne JL, Gattaz F, Guidicelli H: Additive value of thallium single-photon emission computed tomography myocardial imaging for prediction of perioperative events in clinically selected high cardiac risk patients having abdominal aortic surgery. Am J Cardiol 77:143–148, 1996

38. Pauker SG, Kassirer JP: Decision analysis. N Engl J Med 316:250–258, 1987
39. Kassirer JP, Moskowitz AJ, Lau J, Pauker SG: Decision analysis: A progress report. Ann Intern Med 106:275–291, 1987
40. Richardson WS, Detsky AS: Users' guides to the medical literature. VII. How to use a clinical decision analysis. B. What are the results and will they help me in caring for my patients? Evidence-based Medicine Working Group. JAMA 273:1610–1613, 1995
41. Fleisher LA, Skolnick ED, Holroyd KJ, Lehmann HP: Coronary artery revascularization before abdominal aortic aneurysm: A decision analytic approach. Anesth Analg 79:661–669, 1994
42. Mason JJ, Owens DK, Harris RA, Cooke JP, Hlatky MA: The role of coronary angiography and coronary revascularization before noncardiac surgery. JAMA 273:1919–1925, 1995

Dennis T. Mangano

6 | Outcome Studies in Perioperative Medicine: The β-Blockade Trials

BACKGROUND

The Impact of Cardiac Morbidity and Mortality

Of the 30 million patients who undergo noncardiac surgery annually in the United States, approximately 10 million have two or more of the major risk factors for coronary artery disease, and one third of these have defined coronary artery disease.[1,2] As a result, more than 1 million of the 30 million patients undergoing surgery suffer perioperative cardiac complications, including myocardial infarction, unstable angina, heart failure, dysrhythmia, or cardiac death. The added cost to the United States healthcare budget for treatment of these complications in the first year following surgery is estimated to exceed $20 billion annually. Furthermore, because surgical patients tend to be older and sicker, it is expected that perioperative complications and their cost will continue to rise as the general population ages.

Proposed Solutions

Solution of the problem of perioperative cardiac morbidity has been approached by a number of investigators who have identified markers of perioperative myocardial infarction,[3] the relationship between nonfatal in-hospital cardiovascular events following surgery and long-term sur-

Outcome Measurements, edited by Kenneth Tuman. Lippincott Williams & Wilkins, Baltimore © 1999

vival,[4,5] and the potentially[1,3,6–8] reversible physiological events that occur perioperatively and that contribute to such morbidity. Principal among these results is the finding that the occurrence of myocardial ischemia immediately following surgery, with emergence from anesthesia, increases the risk of an in-hospital cardiovascular event—such as myocardial infarction, unstable angina, or cardiac death—more than 9-fold[3] and increases the risk of long-term mortality over the first 2 years by 14- to 20-fold.[4] These findings have focused researchers on the phenomenon of emergence ischemia in high-risk patients, leading to a number of insights. First, the persistently exaggerated sympathetic response to surgery was shown to be associated with substantial increases in heart rate throughout hospitalization.[6] Second, myocardial ischemia is commonly associated with increased heart rate.[6–8] The third insight was the recognition of the hypercoaguable state produced in response to surgery and its potential effects on myocardial ischemia.[6] Finally, endothelial dysfunction, including plaque instability, is precipitated by a variety of perioperative phenomena, including an exaggerated inflammatory response, adding to the previously mentioned excitotoxic response to surgery.[9,10] This complex picture, describing the factors potentially associated with myocardial ischemia infarction, has been recognized for approximately one decade, and investigators have accordingly attempted to ameliorate the impact of such factors in a series of relatively small clinical trials. Included were assessments of the effect of the preoperative and intraoperative use of nitrates,[11,12] β-blockers,[13–15] α_2-agonists,[16–18] and calcium channel blockers[19,20] on hemodynamics and measures of myocardial ischemia. Although several of the preliminary findings were encouraging, these trials did not investigate the effects of such therapies when administered over the entire postoperative hospital stay, including the important emergence period. Even more important, the effects of such intensive therapy on long-term morbidity and mortality (that is, after discharge from the hospital) remained unaddressed.

Although it has been recognized that control of the excitoxic response to surgery is critical, despite use of intensive anesthetic/analgesic techniques, it has not substantively been mitigated in these high-risk patients.

Current Practice

Until 1996, the common practice was that high-risk patients undergoing surgery would receive relatively meticulous attention before and during surgery, but not specifically after surgery.[11–16,19,20] As evidence, despite meticulous preoperative control, heart rate commonly exceeded 50% of the preoperative control over the first several postoperative days to the first week following surgery.[7,8] Although such increases in heart rate may be deleterious in patients with atherosclerotic disease, clinicians did little to control increases in heart rates for fear of precipitating heart failure or bronchospasm with the use of β-blockers. The general standard of care prior to 1996 was to treat postoperative pain, but not increases in heart rate *per se,* unless they were markedly exaggerated (i.e., ≥ 100 bpm). Lesser increases in heart rate, although proportionately large (e.g., 50% of resting heart rate) were not, in fact, ignored,[21,22] even in at-risk patients receiving β-blockers chronically.

THE ATENOLOL TRIAL

In the early 1990s, a clinical therapeutic trial was performed in at-risk patients undergoing noncardiac surgery. It was hypothesized that, in patients who had or were at risk of coronary artery disease, the intensive administration of β-blockers before and after surgery, continuing throughout the period of hospitalization, would decrease mortality and the incidence of serious cardiovascular events during the 2 years after surgery.

The following summarizes the construct of this trial as abstracted from the underlying scientific studies.[21,22]

Patient Selection

On the basis of previous studies, an at-risk population was selected representing approximately one third of the general surgical population or 10 million patients per year in the United States. These patients included those with or at risk of coronary artery disease who were scheduled for noncardiac surgery requiring general anesthesia at the San Francisco Veterans Affairs Medical Center. The presence of coronary artery disease was indicated either by: 1) a previous myocardial infarction; 2) typical angina; or 3) atypical angina with a positive stress test.

Patients were considered at risk of coronary artery disease when they had at least two of the following cardiac risk factors: 1) age ≥ 65 years; 2) hypertension; 3) current cigarette smoking; 4) serum cholesterol concentration ≥ 240 mg/dL (6.2 mmol/L); or 5) diabetes mellitus.

A total of 204 patients who agreed to participate in this study were included; 200 were enrolled and underwent randomization (1 patient withdrew and 3 did not undergo surgery). Ninety-nine were assigned to the atenolol group and 101 to the placebo group.

Method for Atenolol Administration

Using a well established protocol for atenolol administration (ISIS trials), the trial was designed as follows. Prior to induction of anesthesia, patients were randomized to receive either atenolol or placebo. Immediately after surgery and daily throughout their hospital stay (for up to 7 days), patients received atenolol or placebo either intravenously or orally, as described below. The intravenous preparation consisted of two 10-mL syringes, each containing 5 mg of atenolol or placebo. The oral preparation consisted of two 50-mg tablets of atenolol or two placebo tablets.

Study drug was administered 30 minutes prior to surgery in the holding area, based on hemodynamic parameters and clinical symptoms. Study drug was administered if the following conditions were satisfied: 1) heart rate ≥ 55 bpm; 2) systolic blood pressure P ≥ 100 mmHg; and 3) no evidence of congestive heart failure, third-degree heart block, or bronchospasm.

If these criteria were met, the first syringe of study drug was infused over a period of 5 minutes, and the patient observed for an additional 5 minutes and reassessed. If the hemodynamic and clinical conditions described were again satisfied, then the second syringe was administered.

On transfer from the operating room to the recovery room or intensive care unit, study drug was again administered intravenously in the same manner.

On the morning of the first postoperative day and each day thereafter until the patient was discharged from the hospital (up to 7 days), patients received study drug in the matter described for intravenous infusion every 12 hours or once a day orally (if possible), at which time, if the above criteria were satisfied, 50 or 100 mg of atenolol or placebo was given daily. The criteria for oral administration was as follows:

1. if the heart rate was >65 bpm and the systolic blood pressure was >100 mmHg, two tablets of atenolol (total dose of 100 mg) or two tablets of placebo were given orally; or
2. if the heart rate was ≥ 55 bpm but <65 bpm and the systolic blood pressure was ≥ 100 mmHg, one tablet of atenolol or placebo was administered;
3. otherwise, no atenolol or placebo was given.

Clinical care of these patients continued with β-blockers replaced by study drug on the morning of surgery and no other protocol-based restrictions of the anesthetic or surgical technique.

Findings of the Atenolol Trials

Hemodynamics and Myocardial Ischemia

Intraoperative hemodynamics (blood pressure and heart rate) are described in Table 6–1.

Bradycardia was more common in atenolol-treated patients; but tachycardia (heart rate >100 bpm) was less common. However, there was no difference in the incidence of severe bradycardia (heart rate <40 bpm), the number of treatments (atropine) of bradycardia, or hypotension (epinephrine, dopamine, ephedrine, or phenylephrine (Table 6–2).

TABLE 6–1. INTRAOPERATIVE HEMODYNAMIC PARAMETERS

	Atenolol (n = 99)	Placebo (n = 101)	P Value*
Systolic blood pressure <80 mmHg	13	16	0.69
Systolic blood pressure >180 mmHg	32	42	0.19
Diastolic blood pressure <50 mmHg	38	37	0.88
Diastolic blood pressure >100 mmHg	25	31	0.43
Heart rate <40 bpm	4	2	0.44
Heart rate <50 bpm	38	15	0.0002[†]
Heart rate >100 bpm	35	54	0.019[†]

*Fisher's exact test (two-tailed).
[†]Statistically significant at $P \leq 0.05$.

TABLE 6–2. INTRAOPERATIVE CARDIOVASCULAR MEDICATIONS

	Atenolol (n = 99)	Placebo (n = 101)	P Value*
Dopamine	0	1	1.0
Epinephrine	0	1	1.0
Phenylephrine	5	4	0.74
Ephedrine	8	7	0.79
Atropine	2	1	0.61

*Fisher's exact test (two-tailed).

Dysrhythmia

Analysis of perioperative dysrhythmia did not demonstrate significant differences between groups for any measure of ventricular or supraventricular ectopy (Table 6–3).

Myocardial Ischemia

There were differences between the groups in the incidence of myocardial ischemia before surgery. Although the incidence of myocardial ischemia during surgery was reduced by approximately one-third in the atenolol compared with the placebo group, no significance was discerned because of the relatively small sample size (Table 6–4).

During the first week following surgery, however, there was a significant 37% reduction in the incidence of ischemia, which was greatest—50%—in the first 2 days following surgery.

TABLE 6–3. HOLTER-DETECTED ARRHYTHMIAS FOR POSTOPERATIVE DAYS 0–7

	Atenolol (mean)	Placebo (mean)	P Value*
Duration (s)	76,435	78,951	0.12
QRS complexes	88,573	107,819	0.0001†
Ventricular ectopics	824	979	0.61
Supraventricular ectopics	1,234	1,386	0.72
Minimal heart rate (bpm)	50	59	0.0001†
Average heart rate (bpm)	75	87	0.0001†
Maximal heart rate (bpm)	113	130	0.0001†

Data are averages for Postoperative Days 0–7 given for each 24-hour recording period.
*Analysis of variance.
†Statistically significant at $P \leq 0.05$.

TABLE 6–4. INCIDENCE OF HOLTER-DETECTED 1-MM ST DEPRESSION LASTING AT LEAST 1 MINUTE

	Atenolol ($n = 99$)	Placebo ($n = 101$)	P Value*
Preoperatively	13	12	0.79
Operatively	12	18	0.26
Postoperative Days 0–7	24	39	0.03†
Postoperative Days 0–2	17	34	0.008†

*Fisher's exact test (two-tailed)
†Statistically significant at $P \leq 0.05$.

Long-Term Results

In the 2 years following surgery, 30 patients died (15.6% of the 192 patients observed at hospital discharge). Of these deaths, 21 occurred in the placebo group and 9 occurred in the atenolol group—12 versus 4 deaths were related to cardiac causes, respectively. Thus, the overall mortality was 55% lower in the atenolol group ($P = 0.019$), and mortality from cardiac causes was 65% lower ($P = 0.033$). The characteristics of the 30 patients who died are described in Table 6–5.

TABLE 6–5. LONG-TERM DEATHS

Patient	Time to death (days)	Cause of Death
Placebo		
1	19	Massive GI hemorrhage
2	24	*Sudden cardiac death
3	33	*CHF, severe CAD
4	35	*CHF
5	97	*Cardiac arrest
6	112	Acute Bronchopneumonia, COPD
7	162	*Sudden cardiac death
8	185	Adeno CA, colon
9	197	*Acute MI, post PTCA
10	236	*Acute MI
11	303	*Cardiac arrest
12	325	Sepsis
13	328	Small bowel obstruction 2° to CA prostate
14	376	*Acute MI
15	384	Bladder CA
16	517	Sepsis 2° bowel obstruction
17	517	*Cardiac arrest
18	629	Metastatic CA, colon
19	658	*Acute MI, ARDS
20	734	*Post MI CVA
21	755	Peritonitis 2° to perforation of ileum
Atenolol		
1	237	Respiratory failure
2	295	*Ventricular tachycardia
3	327	*Severe CAD, sepsis
4	385	Sepsis, ALS
5	416	Metastatic renal CA
6	481	*CHF post-CABG
7	529	ARDS
8	582	*Severe CAD, lung CA
9	656	Metastatic squamous cell CA, larynx, lung

GI, gastrointestinal; CHF, chronic heart failure, CAD = coronary artery disease; COPD, chronic obstructive pulmonary disease; CA, cancer; MI, myocardial infarction; PTCA, percutaneous transluminal coronary angioplasty; ARDS, adult respiratory distress syndrome; CVA, cardiovascular accident; ALS, acute lateral sclerosis; CABG, coronary artery bypass grafting.
*Cardiac death.

The first death in the atenolol group occurred on Day 237, whereas, the first death in the placebo group occurred on Day 19; by Day 237, 10 deaths had already occurred in the placebo group. Therefore, it appears that the principle effect of atenolol occurred over the first 6–8 months following surgery. This finding is consistent with a previous finding describing the relationship between perioperative events and long-term outcome, with principle effects occurring over 6–8 months in this observational study (Figure 6–1).[4]

The early difference in survival between the groups was observed at 1 year (3 deaths in the atenolol group versus 14 in the placebo group; $P = 0.005$) and at 2 years (9 versus 21; $P = 0.019$). The survival rate was significantly greater in the atenolol group at all times (Figure 6–2).[21]

Atenolol-treated patients surviving to hospital discharge had a significant decrease in the rate of cardiac events compared with the rate in the placebo group within 6 months after surgery (there were no such events in the atenolol group, compared with 12 in the placebo group; $P = <0.001$), a decrease of 67% from the rate in the placebo group within 1 year (7 versus 22 events; $P = 0.003$) and of 48% in the 2 years after surgery (16 versus 32 events; $P = 0.008$). The principal effect of atenolol treatment was evident in the first 6–8 months after surgery; the time from the first event in each group was 6 days for the placebo group, compared with 158 days for the atenolol group. Thereafter, there was no substantial difference between the groups (Figure 6–3).[21]

The relationship between the event rate in the months after surgery was analyzed, with patients separated into those with or without postoperative ischemia in the atenolol and placebo groups, and similar phenomenon was found (Figure 6–4).[22]

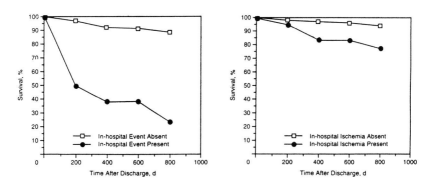

FIGURE 6–1. *Left,* Freedom from cardiac complications after hospital discharge in patients with and without an in-hospital event (postoperative myocardial infarction or unstable angina). *Right,* Freedom from cardiac complications of the hospital discharge in patients with and without postoperative myocardial ischemia detected by ambulatory monitoring.

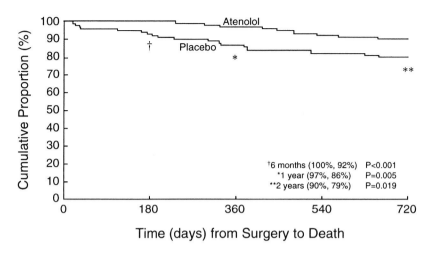

FIGURE 6–2. Survival in the 2 years following surgery.

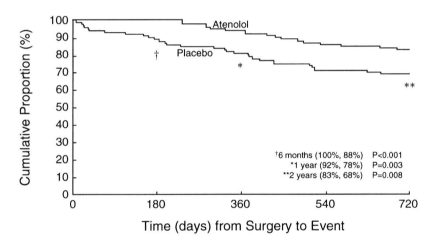

FIGURE 6–3. Event-free survival in the 2 years after noncardiac surgery among 192 patients in the atenolol and placebo groups who survived to hospital discharge.

Other Indicators of Treatment Effect

During treatment, the average heart rate was significantly lower in the atenolol group (75 bpm) versus the placebo group (87 bpm) ($P < 0.001$), as was the maximal heart rate (113 versus 130 bpm; $P < 0.001$).[21] Multivariable correlates associated with survival at 2 years (shown in Table 6–6) were a history of diabetes mellitus and atenolol therapy, with

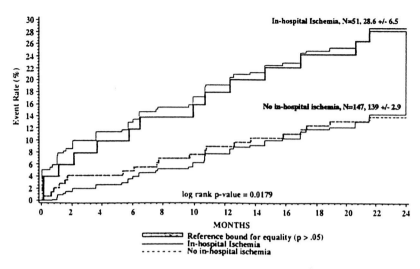

FIGURE 6–4. Atenolol trial overall mortality. Only patients with ischemia on Postoperative Days 0–2 were considered as having in-hospital ischemia.

atenolol improving 2-year survival in patients with diabetes by approximately 75% (hazard ratio for death 0.25; $P = 0.03$).[21] Similarly, in atenolol-treated patients, the presence of diabetes was not associated with a significantly increased risk of death (hazard ratio 1.2; $P = 0.76$), whereas in patients given placebo, the presence of diabetes was associated with a quadrupling of the risk (hazard ratio 4.0; $P = 0.003$). No other perioperative variables were associated with outcome. Several medications were used more frequently in one group than in another, but there was no independent association between the use of these medications and outcome, as shown by the estimated odds ratios and the corresponding P values (Table 6–6).

Tolerance and Adverse Events

During the 2 years after discharge from the hospital, there was no difference between the groups in the use of any cardiovascular medication; therefore, the use of such medications did not confound the observed effects of atenolol on 2-year mortality. These data also indicate that the cardiovascular medications administered before admission to the hospital were still given to most patients at hospital discharge. After discharge, the patients in the placebo group continued to use cardiovascular medications at least as often as the patients in the atenolol group (Table 6–7).

More than 85% of the patients tolerated the intravenous adminis-

TABLE 6-6. PREDICTORS OF DEATH AMONG PATIENTS UNDERGOING NONCARDIAC SURGERY

Predictor	Hazard Ratio (95% CI)	P Value
Univariable models		
Atenolol	0.4 (0.2–0.9)	0.03
Diabetes mellitus	3.1 (1.4–6.8)	0.01
Oral hypoglycemic treatment	2.6 (1.1–6.2)	0.03
Insulin treatment	2.6 (1.0–6.9)	0.05
Ischmia on Holter monitoring on Postoperative Days 0–2	2.3 (1.0–5.3)	0.04
Multivariable models		
Diabetes mellitus	2.8 (1.4–6.2)	0.01
Atenolol	0.5 (0.2–1.1)	0.06

The patients included in these models were the 192 of the original randomized group of 200 who survived to hospital discharge and were followed for 2 years after discharge; 30 of these 192 patients (15.6%) died during the 2 years of follow-up.
CI, confidence interval.

tration of atenolol before surgery and immediately after surgery and its oral administration during the postoperative period; more than 60% were able to receive the full daily dose of atenolol (10 mg intravenously or 100 mg orally) (Table 6–8). In approximately 10% of the patients, the intravenous administration of atenolol before or after surgery was associated with a decrease of ≥20% in the systolic blood pressure or heart rate (Table 6–8); however, no patient had a systolic blood pressure <90 mmHg or a heart rate <40 bpm, and none required therapy. The oral administration of atenolol was not associated with an increased incidence of hypotension, bradycardia, or other event (Table 6–8).

Clinical Implications

The results of this trial indicate that, in patients with or at risk of coronary artery disease undergoing noncardiac surgery, mortality and the incidence of cardiac events after hospital discharge can be reduced by using β-adrenergic blockade throughout the hospital stay. Intensive perioperative β-blockade appears to be safely tolerated, and, given the availability and cost of the generic β-blocking agent, the estimated savings in lives more than outweighs the cost of therapy.

AMERICAN COLLEGE OF PHYSICIANS GUIDELINES

In August 1997, two position papers were published by the American College of Physicians (ACP) defining guidelines for assessing and man-

TABLE 6–7. USE OF CARDIOVASCULAR MEDICATIONS BEFORE AND AFTER SURGERY, ACCORDING TO STUDY GROUP

Study Period	Atenolol n	Placebo n	β-Blockers			Calcium-Channel Blockers			Nitrates			ACE Inhibitors		
			Atenolol	Placebo	P Value	Atenolol	Placebo	P Value	Atenolol	Placebo	P Value	Atenolol	Placebo	P Value
Before admission	99	101	19.4	8.2	0.02[†]	23.7	34.7	0.11[‡]	8.6	13.3	0.36	23.7	8.2	0.003[§]
Hospital discharge	95[∥]	99	14.0	7.1	0.12[π]	19.4	27.6	0.18[**]	7.5	15.3	0.09[††]	20.4	6.1	0.003[‡‡]
6 mo	93	91	13.8	8.3	0.27	19.0	29.9	0.10[§§]	16.1	22.4	0.30	15.2	18.4	0.58
12 mo	90	85	16.7	13.7	0.61	23.8	30.3	0.36	19.1	26.7	0.25	23.8	23.6	0.98
24 mo	84	78	15.5	13.9	0.79	18.8	25.4	0.36	14.1	18.2	0.51	18.1	21.5	0.61

Data are % of patients unless otherwise noted.
χ^2 statistics were used to compare the two groups.
ACE, angiotensin-converting enzyme.
[†]Odds ratio for mortality at 2 years associated with β-blocker use before admission = 0.80 ($P = 0.73$).
[‡]Odds ratio for mortality at 2 years associated with use of calcium-channel blockers before admission = 1.06 ($P = 0.90$).
[§]Odds ratio for mortality at 2 years associated with ACE inhibitor use before admission = 1.45 ($P = 0.50$).
[∥]One patient of the 95 in the atenolol group was not included in these calculations because surgery was delayed for several days after the study drug was given.
[π]Odds ratio for mortality at 2 years associated with β-blocker use at discharge = 0.61 ($P = 0.52$).
[**]Odds ratio for mortality at 2 years associated with use of calcium-channel blockers at discharge = 0.85 ($P = 0.74$).
[††]Odds ratio for mortality at 2 years associated with nitrate use at discharge = 1.32 ($P = 0.64$).
[‡‡]Odds ratio for mortality at 2 years associated with ACE inhibitor use at discharge = 1.17 ($P = 0.79$).
[§§]Odds ratio for mortality at 2 years associated with use of calcium-channel blockers for 6 months = 1.05 ($P = 0.92$).

TABLE 6–8. DAILY DOSE AND SIDE EFFECTS OF ATENOLOL.

Variable	Before Surgery		After Surgery		Days 1–7[†]	
	Atenolol	Placebo	Atenolol	Placebo	Atenolol	Placebo
			(percentage of patients)			
Dosage[‡]						
Full dose	69	79	74	88	63	82
Half dose	19	10	10	6	30	18
Not treated	11	12	15	7	6	1
Side effects						
Hypotension						
Systolic BP <90 mm Hg	0	0	0	0	14	12
>20% decrease in systolic BP	4	0	2	0	—	—
Treated	0	0	0	0	0	0
Bradycardia[§]						
Heart rate <40 bpm	0	0	0	0	6	5
>20% decrease in heart rate	9	0	4	0	—	—
Treated	0	0	0	0	0	0
Bradycardia and hypotension						
Systolic BP <90 mm Hg and heart rate <40 bpm	0	0	0	0	0	0
>20% decrease in heart rate and systolic BP	2	0	1	0	—	—
Treated	0	0	0	0	0	0
Congestive heart failure	0	0	0	0	2	5
Bronchospasm[‖]	3	0	0	0	0	0

$n = 99$ in the atenolol group; $n = 101$ in the placebo groups.
BP, blood pressure.
[*]There were 99 patients in the atenolol group and 101 in the placebo group. BP denotes blood pressure, and bpm beats per minute.
[†]Effects include hypotension, bradycardia, congestive heart failure, or bronchospasm at any time on Days 1–7, as reported by the clinical staff.
[‡]The full dose was 10 mg for intravenous administration, and 100 mg for oral administration. A half-dose was 5 mg intravenously and 50 mg orally. Patients not treated received no study drug because the criteria for administration were not met.
[§]Two patients in the atenolol group whose condition was stable after intravenous drug administration received treatment after intubation for bradycardia 30–75 minutes after the intravenous administration of atenolol.
[‖]Two patients had bronchospasm after intubation, 1 to 3 hours after intravenous atenolol administration; one patient had bronchospasm after extubation, 8.5 hours after intravenous atenolol administration.

aging the perioperative risk from coronary artery disease associated with major noncardiac surgery.[23,24] The first of these articles was titled "Guidelines for Assessing and Managing Perioperative Risk from Coronary Artery Disease Associated with Major Noncardiac Surgery." In this article, the paradigm for management strategy was delineated, and is summarized in Figure 6–5.

The ACP-suggested paradigm regarding use of β-blockers is demonstrated, and the criteria suggested by the ACP were those of Mangano and colleagues.[21] These criteria are: coronary artery disease (defined as a previous myocardial infarction, typical angina, or atypical angina with positive results on a stress test) or risk of coronary artery disease (defined as the presence of at least two of the following: age ≥65 years, hypertension, current smoking, serum cholesterol level ≥240 mg/dL [6.2 mmol/L], and diabetes mellitus). Administration of the drug at each time point requires that the heart rate be ≥55 bpm and that the systolic blood pressure be ≥100 mmHg with no evidence of congestive heart failure, third-degree heart block, or bronchospasm. Patients receive two 5-mg doses of intravenous atenolol, each over 5 minutes beginning 30 minutes before surgery and again immediately after surgery. After surgery, patients are given oral atenolol 100 mg (heart

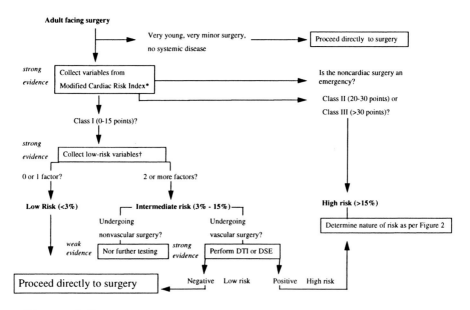

FIGURE 6–5. Suggested algorithm for the risk assessment and management of patients at low or immediate risk of perioperative cardiac events, usually myocardial infarction and death. Boxed phrases indicate recommended actions. Italicized words indicate the level of evidence supporting the recommendation. If there is no word beside the box, there is no evidence for or against its use. DTI, dipridamole-thallium imaging; DSE, dobutamine stress echocardiography.

rate ≥65 bpm) or 50 mg (heart rate 55–64 bpm). If the patient is unable to take oral medication, two 5-mg doses are given intravenously every 12 hours. Atenolol is then given until hospital discharge (maximum 7 days).

The authors' addendum[23] suggested the following:

> In a randomized trial (strong evidence) published after the American College of Physicians reviewed and approved these guidelines, perioperative β-blocker therapy was shown to reduce long-term (6 month) mortality with few side effects. Thus, we recommend the perioperative use of atenolol in patients with coronary artery disease (as per the criteria of Mangano and colleagues), unless the patient has significant contraindications, such as asthma.

In association with the ACP, Palda and Detsky[24] published "Perioperative Assessment and Management Risks from Coronary Artery Surgery," which stated, "Evidence from a randomized, controlled trial has shown a survival benefit with the perioperative use of beta blockers in patients at risk for coronary artery disease." and "High-risk patients need optimum management of their high-risk problems, including beta blocker use . . ."

In their addendum[24], the authors comment:

> Since this background paper and its accompanying guidelines were reviewed by the American College of Physicians, an important publication that we believe should alter current practice has emerged. In December, 1996, the Multicenter Study of Perioperative Ischemia Research Group demonstrated in 200 patients that perioperative β-blockade could substantially reduce mortality rates and rates of nonfatal cardiac events.

and

> We (the authors) believe that this trial is sufficiently convincing, in the absence of contradictory evidence, that it is now appropriate to give atenolol to patients who meet the above criteria, as long as no serious contraindications (such as asthma) are present.

They conclude: "Patients with documented or significant risk factors for coronary artery disease should receive perioperative beta blockade."

Thus, it appears that the ACP has taken a strong position on this issue, marking the first time that any specific perioperative medication has been indicated for the prevention or treatment of cardiovascular complications.

GUIDELINES FOR PERIOPERATIVE BETA BLOCKADE USE

Clearly, given the importance of these findings and the recommendations from the ACP, clinicians must now consider guidelines for perioperative β-blockade use. A number of the guidelines can be synthesized from the recommendations made in these articles, as well from the recommendations of the ACP. Suggested guidelines have evolved from the Multicenter Study of Perioperative Ischemia Research Group,[21,22] and are summarized as follows.

It is recommended that intensive β-blockade be instituted perioperatively in patients with or at risk of coronary artery disease (as previously defined) undergoing noncardiac surgery. Specifically, the standard practice of continuing β-blockers to the time of surgery, when taken chronically, should be continued. However, immediately before surgery, intravenous β-blockade should be instituted according to the suggested protocol to mitigate the effects of emergence tachycardia. Immediately after surgery—in the intensive care unit, the recovery room, or on the ward—the same intensive regimen for administration of intravenous β-blockade should be repeated to mitigate the acute effects of increased heart rate. Thereafter, it is recommended that intensive β-blockade continue intravenously or, if feasible, orally to mitigate the effects of tachycardia during the in-hospital period. A protocol for intravenous or oral administration using a specific β-blocker, atenolol, is shown in Figure 6–6).

CONCLUSIONS

Given the rapid increase in the number of elderly in the world population and the selective admission of older and sicker patients to surgery, it is expected that perioperative cardiovascular morbidity and mortality will continue to increase and consume resources. This serious healthcare problem requires immediate attention. Unfortunately, no therapy had been demonstrated to mitigate in-hospital or longer-term surgical cardiovascular complications. Fortunately, however, recent studies using atenolol have demonstrated that intensive β-blockade, in addition to chronic β-blocker therapy, can mitigate adverse events in the first 6 months following surgery and significantly improve survival. This is the first therapy demonstrated to improve outcome following surgery. Although these studies had focused on a relatively limited population (200 patients), given the evidence for β-blocker effectiveness in patients with ischemic syndromes and the results of surgical observational studies, the findings of this trial are noteworthy. Further, the ACP has taken

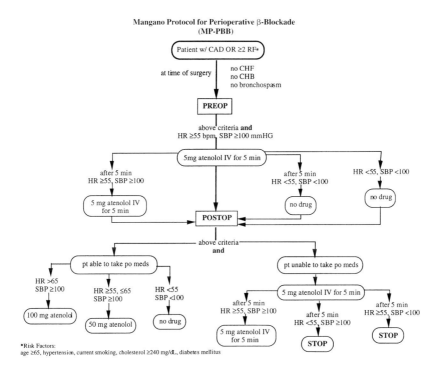

FIGURE 6–6. Atenolol-specific protocol for high-risk patients undergoing non-cardiac surgery.

the bold stand of recommending implementation of perioperative protocols including this therapy. Therefore, clinicians are now, in effect, mandated with the responsibility of developing new perioperative protocols including the intensive use of β-blockade in high-risk patients undergoing surgery.

This therapy appears to have a significant effect on outcome and should be instituted, but it must also be recognized that this is the first of a number of therapies that may have salutary effects. In addition to the phenomena that β-blockade address, including stability of plaque, mitigation of the excitotoxic response, and other salutary effects, therapies addressing other important etiologies for cardiovascular complications also should be considered. Principal among these are therapies that affect platelet adherence, endothelial dysfunction, coronary artery spasm, and other inflammatory and thrombotic phenomena. Therefore, one should view β-blockade as an important, but not complete, therapy for these patients. However, other therapies will only be acceptable if proven by rigorous clinical trials, and when proven, choice of therapy will be dictated by the specific patient profiles. Some patients will require more intensive β-blockade, some antithrombotic agents, and some other newer agents. Further, these therapies may be most effective when extended beyond the hospital stay. Finally, the intensive use of therapies that may modify chronic risk factors such as low-density lipoproteins, should also be considered in these perioperative paradigms.

In summary, aging and surgical selection of sicker patients has mandated that clinicians and clinical researchers address the critical problem of perioperative cardiovascular complications and identify specific therapies for the perioperative environment. The field of perioperative medicine will assume its own identity, thereby enabling integrated and comprehensive approaches to the challenging problems of improving outcome in high-risk patients.

References

1. Mangano D: Perioperative cardiac morbidity. Anesthesiology 72:153–184, 1990
2. Mangano D, Goldman L: Preoperative assessment of patients with known or suspected coronary disease. N Engl J Med 333:1750–1756, 1995
3. Mangano D, Browner W, Hollenberg M, London M, Tubau J, Tateo I, SPI Research Group: Association of perioperative myocardial ischemia with cardiac morbidity and mortality in men undergoing noncardiac surgery. N Engl J Med 323:1781–1788, 1990
4. Mangano D, Browner W, Hollenberg M, Li J, Tateo I, SPI Research Group: Long-term cardiac prognosis following noncardiac surgery. JAMA 268:233–239, 1992
5. Browner W, Li J, Mangano D, SPI Research Group: In-hospital and long-term mortality in male veterans following noncardiac surgery. JAMA 268:228–232, 1992
6. Siliciano D, Mangano D: Postoperative myocardial ischemia: Mechanisms and therapies. In: Estafanous F (ed): Opioids in Anesthesia, pp 164–177. Boston, Butterworth Publishers, 1990
7. Mangano D, Hollenberg M, Fegert G, Meyer M, London M, Tubau J, Krupski W, SPI Research Group: Perioperative myocardial ischemia in patients undergoing noncardiac surgery. I. Incidence and severity during the four-day perioperative period. J Am Coll Cardiol 17:843–850, 1991
8. Mangano D, Wong M, London M, Tubau J, Rapp J, SPI Research Group: Perioperative myocardial ischemia in patients undergoing noncardiac surgery. II. Incidence and severity during the 1st week after surgery. J Am Coll Cardiol 17:851–857, 1991

9. Herskowitz A, Mangano D: The inflammatory cascade: A final common pathway for perioperative injury? Anesthesiology 85:957–960, 1996
10. Hennein H, Ebba H, Rodriguez J, Merrick S, Keith F, Bronstein M, Leung J, Mangano D, Greenfield L, Rankin J: Relationship of the proinflammatory cytokines to myocardial ischemia and dysfunction after uncomplicated coronary revascularization. J Thorac Cardiovasc Surg 108:626–635, 1994
11. Coriat P, Daloz M, Bousseau D, Fusciardi J, Echter E, Viars P: Prevention of intraoperative myocardial ischemia during noncardiac surgery with intravenous nitroglycerin. Anesthesiology 63:193–196, 1984
12. Gallagher J, Moore R, Jose A, Botros S, Clark D: Prophylactic nitroglycerin infusions during coronary artery bypass surgery. Anesthesiology 64:785–789, 1986
13. Stone J, Foëx P, Sear J, Johnson L, Khambatta H, Triner L: Myocardial ischemia in untreated hypertension patients: effect of a single small oral dose of a beta-adrenergic blocking agent. Anesthesiology 68:495–500, 1988
14. Magnusson J, Thulin T, Werner O, Jarhult J, Thomson D: Haemodynamic effects of pretreatment with metropolol in hypertensive patients undergoing surgery. Br J Anaesth 58:251–260, 1986
15. Cucchiara R, Benefiel D, Matteo R, DeWood M, Albin M: Evaluation of esmolol in controlling increases in heart rate and blood pressure during endotracheal intubation in patients undergoing carotid endarterectomy. Anesthesiology 65:528–531, 1986
16. Ghignone M, Calvillo O, Quintin L: Anesthesia and hypertension: The effect of clonidine on perioperative hemodynamics and isoflurane requirements. Anesthesiology 67:3–10, 1987
17. Talke P, Li J, Jain U, Leung JL, Drasner K, Hollenberg M, Mangano D, the SPI Research Group: Effects of perioperative dexmedetomidine infusion in patients undergoing vascular surgery. Anesthesiology 82:620–633, 1995
18. The McSPI—Europe Research Group: Perioperative sympatholysis: Beneficial effects of the α_2 adrenoceptor agonist mivazerol on hemodynamic stability and myocardial ischemia. Anesthesiology 86:346–363, 1997
19. Chung F, Houston P, Cheng D, Lavelle P, McDonald N, Burns R, David T: Calcium channel blockade does not offer adequate protection from perioperative myocardial ischemia. Anesthesiology 69:343–347, 1988
20. Merin R: Calcium channel blocking drugs and anesthetics: Is the drug interaction beneficial or detrimental? Anesthesiology 66:111, 1987

21. Mangano D, Layug E, Wallace A, Tateo I, for the Multicenter Study of Perioperative Ischemia (McSPI) Research Group: Effect of atenolol on mortality and cardiovascular morbidity after noncardiac surgery. N Engl J Med 335:1713–1720, 1996
22. Wallace A, Layug E, Tateo I, Li J, Hollenberg M, Browner W, Miller D, Mangano D, for the Multicenter Study of Perioperative Ischemia (McSPI) Research Group: Prohylactic atenolol reduces postoperative myocardial ischemia. Anesthesiology 88:7–17, 1998
23. The American College of Physicians: Clinical guideline. Part I. Guidelines for assessing and managing the perioperative risk from coronary artery disease associated with major noncardiac surgery. Ann Intern Med 127:309–312, 1997
24. Palda V, Detsky A: Clinical guideline. Part II. Perioperative assessment and management of risk from coronary artery disease. Ann Intern Med 127:313–328, 1997

T. Samuel Shomaker

7 | Practice Guidelines in Cardiovascular Anesthesia

More than 2000 practice guidelines developed by more than 50 different groups, including medical specialty societies and other physician groups, individual hospitals, health maintenance organizations (HMOs), third-party payers, and the federal government have been developed in the United States.[1-4] The extensive effort focused on the development of practice guidelines has resulted in the development of an entirely new body of literature, including manuals on how to develop practice guidelines and publications designed to assist clinicians in the use of these guidelines.[5-11] The investment of large amounts of energy and resources directed toward the development of guidelines aside, there remain many uncertainties regarding practice guidelines. At the most basic level, data are still ambiguous as to whether practice guidelines are really effective in making long-term modifications to physician behavior and, therefore, in controlling healthcare costs.[12] There are also uncertainties in the methodology for harmonizing expert opinion and scientific evidence in guideline development, as well as questions relating to the most effective techniques to influence physicians to use practice guidelines that have already been developed.[13,14] Despite this host of unanswered questions, the philosophical underpinnings of the use of practice guidelines (i.e., standardizing patient care into diagnostic and treatment modalities that have been demonstrated to be scientifically valid and cost-effective will reduce unwarranted and undesirable variations in the use of medical care and limit the cost of medical treatment)

Outcome Measurements, edited by Kenneth Tuman. Lippincott Williams & Wilkins, Baltimore © 1999

make good sense.[15] Practice guidelines have therefore been embraced by many, including the government, third-party payers, and influential specialty groups. These guidelines therefore seem destined to become a permanent fixture in the medical environment of the 21st century.[16] Practice guidelines will be used to influence decisions relative to payment for patient care and the assessment of the quality of medical practice;[17,18] thus, from a practical point of view, a working knowledge of the theory and use of practice guidelines is important for physicians, including cardiovascular anesthesiologists.

Although no comprehensive practice guidelines have been developed for the practice of cardiovascular anesthesia, cardiology and cardiothoracic surgery have seen much activity in the practice guideline area. Guidelines related to specific areas within the practice of cardiothoracic anesthesia, including guidelines for pulmonary artery catheterization[19], echocardiography,[20] and blood component therapy,[21] have been developed by the American Society of Anesthesiologists (ASA). Other guidelines dealing with particular issues in cardiovascular anesthesia have been developed locally or regionally.[22] The Society of Thoracic Surgeons has developed an extensive set of guidelines for the practice of cardiothoracic surgery,[23-31] as has the American College of Cardiology (ACC) in conjunction with the American Heart Association (AHA) for with a wide range of issues in the practice of cardiology.[32-37] A guideline of particular import for cardiovascular anesthesiologists in this series deals with the perioperative cardiovascular evaluation of patients for noncardiac surgery.[34]

Cardiac anesthetists in England, surveyed in October 1994,[38] expressed support for the concept that guidelines are valuable in the practice of medicine (89% versus 6%). However, when asked whether there should be national guidelines for cardiac anesthesia, the cardiac anesthetists were not enthusiastic, with only 21% stating that there should be national guidelines, whereas 69% responded negatively. The stance, taken by most, was not premised on the fact that practice guidelines would be used to establish a standard of care for legal liability or on the inherent technical complexity involved in cardiac anesthesia. Rather, the three most common arguments advanced against the implementation of national guidelines for cardiac anesthesia were:

- That they would fail to reduce irrational variation in clinical practice (this position, the author acknowledged, was somewhat irrational in that the basic premise of guidelines is that they offer a mechanism to tackle the problem of irrational variation of clinical practice). The author maintains that it is not necessarily the drugs or technique used in cardiac anesthesia, but rather the anesthesiologist who is the primary determinant of outcome. The author concedes that if some of

the variation in cardiac anesthesia outcome results from inadequate knowledge or poor skills, then guidelines should help to improve the quality of patient care.
- That the use of guidelines would decrease the flexibility of practitioners and lead to a reduced ability to tailor clinical care to the particular circumstances presented by an individual patient.
- That the adoption of guidelines would not necessarily lead to improved quality of cardiac anesthesia.

The survey results are also interesting for the finding that cardiac anesthetists who worked in institutions in which local guidelines were in place overwhelmingly followed them.

Despite the extensive amount of guideline development efforts in cardiology and cardiothoracic surgery, there is still little in the way of comprehensive guideline development in the area of cardiovascular anesthesia. Whether this is attributable to American cardiac anesthetists adopting similar attitudes to those of their British colleagues or to some other reason(s) is unclear given the current state of the literature.

HISTORY

Practice guidelines are an ancient and time-honored tradition in the practice of medicine. Medical textbooks, from those of ancient vintage to today's modern versions, contain hundreds of generic rules, axioms, treatments, indications, and criteria that can all be considered forms of practice guidelines.[39,40] Consider this approach to the treatment of bronchitis practiced in Syria 3500 years ago:

> If the patient suffers from a hissing cough, if his windpipe is full of murmurs . . . if he has phlegm: braid together roses, and mustard, and purified oil, drop it on his tongue, fill moreover, a tube with it and blow it into his nostrils. Thereafter, he shall drink several times, beer of the first quality: thus he will recover.[41]

Concerns over patient safety sparked the first discussions about proper anesthetic techniques in the 1840s, shortly after the first use of drugs to render patients insensible to pain during operative procedures.[42] These discussions concerned the two most important clinical issues of the day, the relative safety of ether versus chloroform anesthesia and whether the monitoring of pulse and respiration could help to prevent death under anesthesia.[43] John Snow, who was one of the most prominent anesthesiologists of his day, published an article on the fatal cases of inhalation of chloroform in 1849, in which he discussed a number of suggestions to improve the outcomes of patients undergoing surgery under anesthesia.[44] Discussions relating to patient safety in anesthesia continued throughout the remainder of the 19th century as other prominent anesthesiologists joined the debate and provided their suggestions for improving patient care.[45]

The ASA, founded in 1905, has carried on the work of these pioneering anesthesiologists. In the early decades of the 20th century, the ASA conducted studies on anesthetic morbidity and mortality.[42] In 1968, the ASA published one of the earliest documents specifically referred to as a guideline. In keeping with its historic emphasis on patient safety, the Guidelines for Patient Care in Anesthesiology establishes expectations for the quality and type of anesthetic care that each patient should receive in the operating room.[46] It places affirmative obligations on the anesthesiologist to 1) adequately evaluate the patient preoperatively; 2) provide comprehensive care for the patient intraoperatively, including rendering the patient insensitive to pain and monitoring and supporting the patient's vital functions during anesthesia; and 3) provide responsible postanesthetic care.

From this beginning, the ASA has published numerous guidelines on diverse subjects, such as continuing education,[47] critical care,[48] the delineation of clinical privileges,[49] pulmonary artery catheterization,[19] ambulatory surgery facilities,[50] preanesthetic care,[51] peer review,[52] postanesthetic care,[53] blood component therapy,[21] acute pain management,[54] and basic intraoperative monitoring.[55]

The standard on intraoperative monitoring was first issued in 1986 and has become one of the most influential practice standards ever published.[40] The standard adopted by the ASA was modeled on anesthesia monitoring standards in existence at Harvard University.[56] Eichhorn et al.[56] credited the use of the standards to a decreased number of intraoperative complications and a reduction in the department's malpractice liability exposure. When first issued, the standards called for the routine use of an electrocardiogram, blood pressure device, and oxygen sensor.

In the late 1980s, the ASA recognized that the use of pulse oximetry had become a *de facto* standard of care in patient monitoring. Therefore, in 1990, the society formally amended the basic intraoperative monitoring standards to add a requirement for pulse oximetry.[55] It also expanded the standard to obligate anesthetists to verify ventilation, which, in effect, mandated the use of end-tidal capnography to confirm endotracheal tube placement.[55] The standard for intraoperative monitoring is frequently offered as evidence of the effectiveness of practice policies in improving patient care outcomes.[1,57,58] However, even after nearly a decade of experience with the requirement for the use of pulse oximetry and capnography, there is still debate within the anesthesia community about the effectiveness of these monitoring modalities in improving patient outcome and as to whether the adoption of the practice standard truly influenced practitioners to use these monitors or merely codified existing practice.[59,60]

In the area of cardiothoracic anesthesia, the ASA issued its practice guidelines for pulmonary artery catheterization in 1993[19] and in 1996 published practice guidelines for blood component therapy[21] and transesophageal echocardiography.[20] However, the ASA's activity in this field was predated by both the Society of Thoracic Surgeons and the ACC/AHA, which have actively published guidelines in the area of cardiovascular medicine for a number of years. The ACC/AHA task force on practice guidelines was first convened in 1980, and this group has subsequently produced guidelines for a number of areas in cardiovascular medicine, such as preoperative cardiovascular evaluation for noncardiac surgery,[34] evaluation and management of heart failure,[33] clinical application of echocardiography,[36] management of acute myocardial infarction,[35] exercise testing,[37] and clinical intracardiac electrophysiological and catheter ablation procedures.[32]

The Society of Thoracic Surgeons constituted its *ad hoc* committee for cardiothoracic surgical practice guidelines in 1989. This group has gone on to write guidelines in the following areas of thoracic surgery: ischemic heart disease;[25] valvular heart disease;[30] thoracic aortic disease;[29] chest wall, diaphragm, mediastinum, and pericardium;[23] esophageal disease;[24] bronchopulmonary disease;[26] transplantation and heart assist devices;[28] electrical problems;[29] and congenital heart disease.[27] These and other guidelines relevant to cardiac anesthesia are discussed in detail later in this chapter.

DEFINITIONS

Practice guidelines are "developed by a formal process that incorporates the best scientific evidence with expert opinion"[61] and are "systematically developed statements to assist practitioner and patient decisions about appropriate health care for specific clinical circumstances."[62] Guidelines are intended to be a flexible tool that can be used to assist practitioners in the management of particular clinical conditions. Therefore, they can be adopted, modified, or rejected according to clinical needs and constraints. Many other terms have also been coined to describe similar instruments formatted to assist the process of patient care. These include:

- practice policies describe preset recommendations issued to influence practitioners in reaching decisions about healthcare interventions.[3]
- protocols and algorithms are stepwise procedures or decision trees used to guide practitioners through the diagnosis and treatment of various clinical problems.[64]

- parameter is a term that the American Medical Association (AMA) originated, which is defined as a generic term for "acceptable approaches to the prevention, diagnosis, treatment or management of disease or condition, as determined by the medical profession based on the best medical evidence currently available."[65]

Guidelines, practice policies, protocols, and parameters are all voluntary guides used to assist the physician in patient management. They can be adopted verbatim, modified, or rejected as the clinician sees fit and as the circumstances of the case dictate.

Standards of care, although closely related to guidelines, are different in intent and effect. A standard of care is an authoritative statement that establishes minimal levels of acceptable performance.[66] According to Eddy,[66] practice standards are justified when the health and economic consequences of an intervention are very well known and when unanimity exists among patients about the desirability of the intervention and among physicians about the proper use of the intervention. Practice standards therefore carry an air of compulsion and are more rigidly applied. For legal purposes, practice standards establish the relevant standard of care to which practitioners must conform.[67,68] Failure to follow an established practice standard is often held to be an admission that the clinical care rendered to a patient is legally inadequate.[69,70] Most of the clinical decision aids that have been published are ostensibly guidelines rather than practice standards, but even guidelines and protocols are often interpreted as establishing the relevant standard of care in medical malpractice cases related to the subject matter that they cover. This is true even though many guidelines contain specific disclaimers intended to prevent their use in this way.[71] For example, the disclaimer contained in the ASA Practice Guidelines for Pulmonary Artery Catheterization states: " . . . these recommendations are intended as general guidelines. Departure from these guidelines should not necessarily be viewed as inappropriate care."[19] A similar disclaimer is contained in the ACC/AHA series of guidelines, which states:

> These practice guidelines are intended to assist physicians in clinical decision making by describing a range of generally acceptable approaches for the diagnosis, management, or prevention of specific diseases or conditions. These guidelines attempt to define practices that meet the needs of most patients in most circumstances. The ultimate decision must be made by the physician and the patient in light of all the circumstances presented by the patient.[35]

Despite these statements, which are intended to discourage the broad adoption of guidelines as standards of care, the existence of practice guidelines has proved decisive in a number of legal cases, either for the plaintiff, arguing that the treating physician failed to follow an established practice guideline,[69,70] or for the defendant, alleging that the physician followed a practice guideline and thus was not liable.[68]

WHY ARE PRACTICE GUIDELINES NEEDED?

The notion of evidence-based medicine, i.e., that the use of diagnostic and treatment modalities should be based on evidence of effectiveness as determined in scientific trials contained in the medical literature, is now gaining currency.[72,73] Developments in this area have been made far more practical for day to day use in physician practices by information management software developed only recently.[74,75] However, it remains true today—and was truer still 10 years ago—that much of what is advocated in medical textbooks is based on anecdotal experience, not on formally obtained scientific evidence. This was recognized in the early 1970s by Cochrane[76], a British physician who advocated the use of randomized, controlled, clinical trials to guide decisions about healthcare as an alternative to the nonscientific evidentiary foundation of many medical decisions of the day. Although many medical schools are now moving to change educational practice in this area, most physicians in training are still not taught to critically read the medical literature and apply the evidence obtained to the management of individual patient cases.[77,78] The inadequate state and use of the scientific foundation of medicine is one factor in the tremendous variability in care provided to patients with similar conditions that has been shown by many recent studies.[79–84] With the lack of evidence-based medicine, these variations in patient care are viewed with suspicion by physicians, patients, and third-party payers. Indeed, a number of recent studies have placed the number of procedures performed for inappropriate indications at 10%–30%.[59] This does not take into consideration patient intervention, diagnostic tests, or treatment modalities that are used despite little or no demonstrated efficacy. Inappropriate or nonefficacious procedures add greatly to the cost of healthcare in the United States.[40,63]

The recent preoccupation with guidelines is one byproduct of the growing concern about rising healthcare costs in the United States. As one author states, "U.S. healthcare policy makers and payers have seized on guidelines as a 'magic bullet' for eliminating presumably unnecessary care and its associated costs."[16] Although guidelines play a role in cost-containment, viewing them as panacea is far too simplistic an approach. Clinical practice guidelines are at the foundation of the managed care revolution that has swept the healthcare system in the United States over the past 5 years. Through the twin processes of clinical practice guideline establishment and utilization review, managed care organizations have sought to steer clinical practice into certain clinical patient management strategies that they believe are of proven efficacy in an attempt to reduce unnecessary care and its associated costs while maintaining healthcare quality.[4,64] The Institute of Medicine and the National Academy of Sciences listed a number of important roles that guidelines can play in the healthcare system of the 21st century.[5] These are:

- cost control: there is evidence that guidelines, when rationally designed, can contribute to controlling healthcare costs.
- quality assurance: if guidelines can limit the use of treatment modalities of little or no efficacy and decrease the patient's exposure to the risk that these procedures entail, healthcare quality will improve.
- enhancing access to care: if guidelines can reduce unnecessary care, they will free resources to extend healthcare services to more people.
- patient empowerment: patients more and more want to be involved as partners in decisions affecting their healthcare. It is incumbent on providers to communicate information to consumers more effectively so that they can make informed choices. To the extent that guidelines can reduce uncertainty and make implicit assumptions explicit, placing this type of information in the hands of consumers will assist in improving the healthcare market.
- professional autonomy and medical liability: some physician organizations see guidelines as an opportunity to maintain control over their own destiny. By promulgating guidelines themselves, they reduce the chance of having guidelines imposed on them from outside. As a collary to this consideration, the formulation of guidelines by professional societies can limit exposure to medical malpractice liability.

Another physician has proposed a series of alternative goals for the use of practice guidelines:[16] 1) to assess and ensure quality of care by assisting clinical decision-making by patients and practitioners through a reduction of uncertainty and by educating the public individually or in groups; 2) to guide the allocation of resources for healthcare, particularly at the level of practitioners and institutions; 3) to reduce the risk of negligent care and ensuing liability.

Despite the seemingly compelling arguments for the formulation and adoption of well researched clinical practice guidelines, there is a great deal of debate within the medical field itself about the relative advantages and disadvantages of the use of practice guidelines.[4] Critics maintain that clinical practice guidelines can not be written in enough detail to account for the myriad of possible clinical scenarios. It has been argued that forcing practitioners to use clinical practice guidelines robs them of their professional autonomy, which is so important in providing quality patient care, and leads to the practice of "cookbook medicine."[4] In fact, these critics argue that the intensive loss of professional autonomy may ultimately affect the quality of the profession overall, as the attractiveness of medicine as a career will decline if a physician's ability to exercise independent judgment is substantially curtailed. Critics also contend that heavy reliance on practice guidelines may discourage technical innovation and trail-breaking research because experimentation with new technologies may not be considered under existing practice guidelines.[85,86] This is particularly true if guidelines are made the standard of medical care, because failure to follow practice guidelines will, in those cases, potentially lead to more liability on the part of physicians who depart from the guidelines in caring for patients.[87,88] This may be true even in situations in which physicians have good reasons for not following practice guidelines. Finally, despite a wealth of speculation about the potential effects guidelines can have on constraining healthcare costs, there are no definitive data to suggest that the use of guidelines is cost-effective, especially when factoring in the cost of developing, publicizing, and implementing practice guidelines.

Many in the medical community, however, welcome the advent of practice guidelines as the profession's best hope for accommodating the competing demands for quality healthcare at the lowest possible price.[39] Those in this camp view guidelines as a time-saving adjunct to the already complex task of medical decision-making. As Eddy[39] observed:

> Practice policies present a powerful solution to the complexities of medical decisions. They free practitioners from the burden of having to estimate and weigh the pros and cons of each decision. They can connect each practitioner to a collective consciousness, bringing order, direction and consistency to their decisions. Practice policies provide an intellectual vehicle through which the profession can bestow the lessons of research in clinical experiences and put the knowledge and preferences of many people into conclusions about appropriate practices. They provide a natural pathway to convey that information to practitioners. Practice policies are the central nervous system of medical practice.[39]

It can be assumed that all physicians want to deliver healthcare of the highest possible quality at the lowest possible cost, and, as one practitioner has observed, practice guidelines can assist in this endeavor because they are "in effect what the clinician would create personally if he or she had the time and resources to accomplish a full evaluation alone ... guidelines summarize the collective as determined scientifically."[63]

One of the traditional objections to the use of practice guidelines and evidence-based medicine in general is the cumbersome nature of attempting to find and apply guidelines and other medical literature to a particular patient's situation, given the time constraints of modern medical practice. The advent of the electronic medical records may make concerns of this kind obsolete. Programming for the electronic medical record can be written so that clinical practice guidelines and practice tips, along with drug interaction warnings and other clinical data, can be furnished to clinicians in real time, as they care for a patient during a clinic or hospital visit.[89] These emerging technologies argue even more strongly for the fact that clinical practice guidelines will become a long-term fixture in the practice of medicine.

DEVELOPMENT THROUGH THE YEARS

Many organizations have developed practice guidelines, and there are a large number of new entrants in the field every year. The list includes the Agency for Healthcare Policy Research (AHCPR) at the federal level,[40] a large number of medical specialty societies,[65] national medical organizations such as the AMA and the Academic Medical Center Consortium,[1] third-party payers such as insurance companies[88] or HMOs,[64] and individual hospitals or local provider groups.[90–92] The approach that the organization writing the practice policy uses depends on the underlying objectives of the group.[93,94] For example, healthcare cost-containment is the primary motivating factor for third-party payers and HMOs who engage in the process of clinical guideline development. On the other hand, national organizations such as the AMA and the AHCPR have stated their objectives in the guideline development process to be the improvement of the quality of patient care in medical practice. Obviously, to the user of a guideline, the quality of content is the primary consideration. However, users must bear in mind that the perspective taken by the developing group can subtly bias even quality guidelines. Therefore, medical practitioners must be aware of and sensitive to the potential for this type of influence.

Although different groups write guidelines for different reasons, there is a consensus on the attributes that quality practice guidelines should contain. In its publication Guidelines for Clinical Practice: From Development to Use,[5] the Institute of Medicine has established criteria for evaluating the effectiveness of practice guidelines. The characteristics emphasized include validity, strength of evidence, reliability, applicability, flexibility, clarity, a well planned development process, and provisions for regular review and revision.

There are a number of books written about the methodology for developing practice guidelines.[2,3,5] Eddy[95] identified five main objectives that the methodology should strive to satisfy:

First, the method should produce policies that are accurate. The outcomes actually affected by the policies should be outcomes that the people who design the policies think they are influencing. Second, the method should be accountable, enabling others to review the reasoning behind the policy. Third, it should enable people to anticipate the health and financial consequences of applying a policy both to an individual and to a population. Fourth, the method should facilitate resolution of conflicts across policies. Finally, it should facilitate the application of the policy, both to individual patients and to populations.[11]

These objectives attempt to ensure that the policy is accurate, accountable, predictable, defensible, and usable. Three examples of guideline development methodology are now discussed.

The Consensus Development Program was begun by the National Institutes of Health (NIH) in 1977 and has analyzed more than 60 clinical topics to date.[96] Topics are selected in areas in which there are considerable clinical controversy and uncertainty. The objective of the process is to reach a consensus as to the appropriate approach to take to clinical questions arising in these areas. The process is initiated with the selection of a clinical topic. NIH staff then performs an extensive data search to select the most current medical literature that pertains to the selected topic. A panel of experts consisting of scientists, physicians, and informed laypersons are selected by NIH to review these scientific data. As a result of the initial review, a list of questions posed by the topic is constructed. A 2-day executive session is then convened, at which the expert panel attempts to reach a consensus on the issues posed. As an outgrowth of this executive session, a consensus document that contains one or more specific recommendations or clinical guidelines is prepared. This document is then circulated among the community of practicing physicians.

Another example of guideline development methodology is the process used to develop the AHCPR guideline on unstable angina.[97] The development methodology used in this case is similar to that employed in the formulation of other AHCPR guidelines. An expert panel is convened and supported by AHCPR. In other AHCPR guidelines, private contractors are used in the process of guideline development. For example, the guideline developed under the auspices of AHCPR on cardiac rehabilitation was developed under a contract with the American Association of Cardiovascular and Pulmonary Rehabilitation.[98] The unstable angina guideline was formulated by an expert panel consisting of cardiologists; cardiac surgeons; emergency medicine, family medicine, and internal medicine physicians; cardiac nurses; and consumer and public health representatives. In preparation for the panel's work, staff performed a literature search, which revealed an extensive bibliography containing more than 5000 abstracts relating to the general subject of unstable angina. The abstracts were reviewed, and 2500 relevant articles were selected and organized using an outline of topics relating to the customary management of patients with angina. The staff then reviewed the 2500 relevant abstracts and selected 130 randomized clinical trials, 319 clinical studies of excellent quality, and 1351 clinical studies of good quality, all of which were reviewed for appropriateness of methodology and summarized for the panel's use. In general, only published articles were used in the panel's deliberation; however, a small number of unpublished randomized trials that had been presented at scientific meetings were reviewed and summarized for use by the panel.

Studies that related to a particular guideline recommendation made by the panel were reviewed together to assess the overall strength of the scientific evidence available to support the recommendation. Strength of evidence was rated A if the overall quality and consistency of the literature supporting the recommendation were strong and there was at least one randomized controlled trial included as part of the data. Evidence was rated B if there were well conducted clinical studies available but no randomized clinical trials on the topic under consideration. A grade of C was given for cases in which there was a dearth of relevant clinical studies of good quality. The panel assessed the strength of evidence, and an informal process of group discussion was used to achieve consensus on the language of each recommendation and the strength of the evidence supporting it. The panel found little or no evidence to assist its deliberation on many issues in the area of the diagnosis and management of angina. The panel also noted that there was no necessary relationship between the clinical substantiveness of a particular topic and the availability and significance of the scientific evidence relating to that topic. In areas in which little or no evidentiary material was available, expert opinion was used as a guide to formulate recommendations. Each recommendation was modified by an assessment of the scientific evidence available to support the recommendation. For example, one of the panel's recommendations relates to entry into medical care with patients suspected to have unstable angina. It reads:

> recommendation: because both clinical examination and ECG are critical to early risk assessment, the initial evaluation of a patient with symptoms suggesting possible unstable angina, should be done by a medical practitioner in a facility equipped to perform an ECG and not over the telephone (strength of evidence = B).[97]

Each recommendation is then followed by a description of the panel's rationale and an assessment of the documentation available to support the recommendation.

Before finalizing the recommendations, the guidelines were revised to reflect the comments of a number of individuals representing 24 professional peer organizations with expertise in the area of unstable angina. It was then reviewed and tested by 44 practitioners who assessed whether the document was practical and reasonable for use in clinical practice.

Yet another methodology, developed by Browman et al.,[90] illustrates another approach to guideline development that may be more rigorous than that used by the AHCPR. This cycle involves an eight-step development process starting with the identification of a clinical problem to be investigated. Next, recommendations are generated based on consideration of the scientific evidence available to support the guideline. This step involves searching existing guidelines, gathering and synthesizing available evidence, grading the strength of the evidence obtained, and generating preliminary evidence-based recommendation(s). Unfortunately, as in the AHCPR development process, randomized clinical trials, which are the gold standard of scientific evidence, are rarely available; even when they can be identified, trials are often limited in scope and do not cover the complete range of situations that a practice guideline is intended to address.[61,99] A 1987 publication illustrated the magnitude of the issues in this area.[100] The article attempted to review the scientific literature to define the appropriate indications for six common clinical procedures. Of the articles relevant to the topics, only 10% were randomized controlled trials, and more than two-thirds were retrospective studies. In most cases, the information on the indications for or the efficacy of the procedures was either incomplete or contradictory. Given the limitations of the available data, less specific relevant information must often be considered. Despite this reality, it is still important to use some organized mechanism to grade the strength of evidence used in constructing the practice guideline.[99,101–104]

Step three in the Browman et al. methodology is to have an expert group reconcile the various data contained in the available evidence to arrive at a final recommendation. In the fourth step, modulating factors are applied to the scientific data. This step is important to build clinical flexibility into the guidelines, as well as to introduce significant variables that may influence the use on the guideline in practice, such as cost-benefit information and patient preference.[105] The next step, independent review, is important to increase the credibility and legitimacy of the guideline. A number of independent experts who have had no hand in the development process are used to fulfill this function. The subsequent phase is to formulate a plan for the administrative implementation of the guideline. This includes a plan for the dissemination of and tracking the use of the guideline. Once the guideline has been officially approved by the sponsoring organization, it is then disseminated and put into practice. The eighth and final step in the process is the establishment of a mechanism for reviewing and updating the guideline on a regular basis to account for new knowledge in the area.

DISSEMINATION

An important but often overlooked issue in the usefulness of a clinical practice guideline is how the guideline is put into the hands of those who are expected to use it.[13,93] Even a well formulated guideline is of little use unless it reaches its intended target audience. Interested audiences may include healthcare practitioners, consumers, the healthcare industry, health policy makers, researchers, and the media. The AHCPR has considered the issue of guideline dissemination in depth and has formulated a series of strategies for getting information about guidelines to intended consumers.[106,107] In addition to efforts intended to publicize the particular guidelines AHCPR develops, the agency also develops audience-specific products. For example, in addition to the full guideline document, which contains the technical description of the guideline, its scientific basis, an explanation of the methodology, and complete documentation relating to the references used in development, the agency also published three other documents:[107] the clinical practice guideline, which contains the complete guideline with recommendations and references pertinent to the recommendations; the quick reference guide, which has key findings and recommendations from the guideline and is intended for quick use in the healthcare setting; and a consumer version, which is patient-centered and is intended to provide information to patients so that they may be better informed.

As an illustration of the strategies employed on the introduction of a new AHCPR guideline, the example of the acute pain management guideline, released on March 5, 1992, by the Secretary of the Department of Health and Human Services (DHHS), is instructive. The guideline was introduced at a press conference sponsored by DHHS on March 5. Participating in this press conference were organizations that had contributed to the formulation of the guideline, including representatives from the AMA, the American Nurses Association, the American Academy of Pain Management, and the American Pain Society. Advance work with the press helped to ensure that news of the guideline made the front page of 11 newspapers across the country. It was also covered widely by television broadcast news reports. The active publicity efforts of the AHCPR ensured that, as of October 19, 1992, the pain guideline had been highlighted in more than 1000 news stories, 12 trade press publications, and 5 journals.[107] The guideline was also made available on electronic databases both at the National Library of Medicine and the National Technical Information Service.

IMPLEMENTATION

Once a guideline has been formulated and disseminated, the next crucial step in securing the guideline's use in practice is to ensure that it becomes assimilated into the daily practice of individual physicians. Many obstacles can interfere with even the best planned efforts to get relevant evidence into the hands of practicing physicians. Hanes[99] highlighted some of the problems that crop up in the process of applying evidence-based medicine to the clinical care of patients. The first obstacle in dealing with a patient management problem is difficulty in finding clinically relevant evidence. As previously discussed, there may be very little published on a particular aspect of a clinical situation. Many physicians lack the training that they need in informatics to search the medical literature and obtain the available evidence.[108,109] Even those who can obtain the evidence sometimes find it difficult to evaluate the validity of the information because specific training in literature analysis has not, until recently, been a traditional part of medical education.[72] Finally, even if evidence is available in the literature, it is unlikely that a busy clinician will have the time to find the evidence and immediately use it to care for the patient.[109]

Some of the problems posed by the state of medical evidence can be overcome by the development of practice guidelines, which summarize the available evidence and may be more readily available than the original literature.[99] This is especially true today with the advent of the electronic medical record, which can be designed so that data entered about a particular patient and diagnosis can prompt the display of relevant practice guidelines, which can then be used to formulate a plan for the diagnosis and therapy of a particular patient's problem.[89]

However, there are difficulties even in areas for which practice guidelines have been formulated. As previously mentioned, guidelines are available only for a small fraction of the clinical conditions encountered by practitioners.[40,61] Furthermore, the particular nuances of patient's symptoms may make it difficult for a practitioner to fit them into an available practice guideline. In addition, there are even instances in which clinical practice guidelines developed by different organizations and using different methodologies conflict in their recommendations. This places the practitioner in an awkward position and leads to reluctance to use clinical practice guidelines.[93,110]

Breast cancer screening is an example of this type of controversy.[111] In 1980, the American Cancer Society recommended that women aged 40–49 years undergo an annual mammogram.[112] This recommendation was made despite the lack of definitive data reflecting the effectiveness of an intervention of this type in that particular age group. Nevertheless, this advice gradually became incorporated into the cancer prevention guidelines of most major organizations involved in cancer treatment, including the National Cancer Institute,[113] the AMA,[114] the American College of Obstetricians and Gynecologists,[115] and the American College of Radiology.[116] In 1993, a study reviewed the available data,[117] including eight major randomized controlled trials of breast cancer screening, as well as a meta-analysis of six of those trials. It concluded that screening for women aged ≥50 years was supported by the literature, but that screening in the 40–49 age group was not linked with a statistically significant effect on mortality. The National Cancer Institute proposed new guidelines based on this study, which recommended that women aged 40–49 years be screened only if they have certain risk factors for the development of breast cancer.[118] Although this position was also advocated by the American Academy of Family Physicians,[119] the American College of Physicians,[120] and the United States Preventive Services Task Force,[121] a storm of protest was generated by patient advocacy groups, medical organizations, and the American Cancer Society. Accordingly, the National Cancer Institute rejected the proposed changes to the cancer screening guidelines.[122] It is conflict of this type that has led some to call for a national clearinghouse on practice guidelines that would have the responsibility of screening available guidelines, analyzing their methodology and evidentiary foundation, and reconciling conflicts. In fact, such a clearinghouse is set to be established under the auspices of AHCPR.[123]

It has proven difficult to influence medical caregivers to change their behaviors to conform with recommendations contained in practice guidelines using traditional approaches such as continuing medical education, financial incentives, and even the threat of legal liability.[124–126] Other techniques have been used to better effect and appear to work in certain circumstances. Under some conditions, guidelines geared to local conditions have been better accepted by practitioners than nationally promulgated guidelines.[93,127–129] Giving physicians a stake in the guideline-writing process has also proved to be an effective approach in helping to collect support for particular guidelines.[1,130,131] However, the most effective techniques have involved the use of peer pressure.[92,131–135] Social influence techniques use a combination of information transfer and the pressure of professional norms, values, and behaviors to convince practitioners to change their practice behavior. These techniques have been applied in various settings, including individual educational settings and moderate to large group meetings. These techniques rely on the premise that individual practitioners can be influenced by the demonstration that their practices fall outside of the norms accepted by their peer group. Examples include the use of one-on-one educational encounters,[136] group meetings with opinion leaders,[137] or participation in quality improvement processes in which cases are discussed and guidelines are used.[138]

ARE PRACTICE GUIDELINES EFFECTIVE?

The effectiveness of practice guidelines is a hotly debated and unresolved question. Outcome studies have reached different conclusions in different settings.[1,10,124–126,128,129] On one hand, some studies demonstrate that practice parameters can be effective in altering physician behavior. For example, one study demonstrated that the adoption of a practice guideline concerning the appropriate use of cesarean sections decreased cesarean section rates while maintaining steady levels of fetal and maternal morbidity and mortality.[139] A hospital seeking to improve the efficiency of usage of critical care resources demonstrated substantial declines in the usage of pacemakers[65] and more rapid transfer of cardiac patients out of coronary care units subsequent to the adoption of a guideline dealing with the appropriate usage of cardiac pacemaking.[140] A guideline on the proper timing of prophylactic antibiotic administration during the perioperative period corresponded with a 50% decline in the incidence of postoperative wound infection.[141] A guideline related to the appropriate transfusion of platelets demonstrated improved blood transfusion practice in a university hospital.[142] A guideline relating to the appropriate usage of costly anesthetics was effective in lowering pharmaceutical costs.[143] In addition, the monitoring standards developed by the ASA, which were discussed earlier, are also advanced as evidence for the effectiveness of practice guidelines.[54,144] However, despite these examples, it is still unclear whether the improvements noted in physician practice behavior are sustained over time.

On the other hand are studies that suggest that practice guidelines have no lasting impact on clinical practice and even less of an effect on improving patient health.[10,124,125] Several studies suggest that many clinicians feel that guidelines are an abridgment of their clinical autonomy and do not account for the reality of today's time-pressured clinical practice.[111,126] Clearly, given the current controversy in the literature over the effectiveness of guidelines, many unanswered questions remain. It seems clear that guidelines are here to stay, but only time and further study will reveal whether guidelines can deliver on their promise of improving clinical practice.

CARDIAC CARE GUIDELINES

A number of guidelines that deal with subjects in the area of cardiac care have been written. These include guidelines authored by the ASA,[19–21] the ACC,[32–37] the Society of Thoracic Surgeons,[23–31] and the AHCPR.[97,98,145,146] However, none of these guidelines deal directly with cardiac anesthesia. Despite all of the activity in the fields of cardiology and thoracic surgery in the area of guideline development, no national organization has taken on the task of writing protocols to guide the practice of cardiac anesthesia.

Some of the guidelines written by organizations with practitioners involved in the care of cardiac patients are applicable to cardiac anesthesia. For example, the ASA has written four guidelines that affect aspects of the practice of cardiac anesthesia, one of which[20] was written in conjunction with the Society of Cardiovascular Anesthesiologists. Others include Practice Guidelines for Blood Component Therapy,[21] Practice Guidelines for Acute Pain Management in the Perioperative Setting,[54] and Practice Guidelines for Pulmonary Artery Catheterization.[19]

The pain management guideline focuses primarily on the process of pain management, rather than on specific pain management techniques or pharmacology.[54] Twelve recommendations were made by the guidelines, as follows:

- An individualized, proactive pain management plan should be established for all surgical patients.
- Hospital personnel should be trained in pain management procedures to reduce the risk of adverse effects.
- Patients and family should be educated about and participate in perioperative pain control.
- The assessment and management of perioperative pain should be documented as part of the patient's record.
- Anesthesiologists trained in pain management should be available 24 hours per day.
- Standard institutional policies for ordering, administering, discontinuing, and transferring responsibility for pain management should be in place.
- Three specific techniques were recognized as particularly effective in the control of perioperative pain: patient-controlled analgesia (PCA) with systemic opioids, epidural analgesia with opioids and/or opioid-local anesthetic mixtures, and regional anesthetic techniques.
- The literature suggests that combinations of analgesic techniques are more effective than single techniques in the control of perioperative pain.
- An organized interdisciplinary approach should be used in pain management.
- Pediatric pain problems present special recognition and management features.
- Geriatric patient populations also have specific pain management issues.
- Patients undergoing ambulatory surgery require special consideration.

The guideline also includes suggestions about information to be included in pain management flow sheets, PCA and epidural analgesia orders, and daily assessment of patients treated with PCA, opioids, and epidural analgesics. The guideline also contains an assessment of the cost of implementing the recommendations, which was estimated at $3705 by a panel of 61 consultant anesthesiologists with expertise in pain management. The guideline does not deal with thoracic epidural analgesia, but a number of the techniques described may relate to strategies that could be employed in the care of patients undergoing cardiac or thoracic surgery.

A second interesting guideline issued by the ASA is the guideline relating to pulmonary artery catheterization,[19] which illustrates some of the difficulties encountered in the development of these tools. Although a panel of experts reviewed more than 860 articles that dealt with pulmonary artery catheterization, a lack of conclusive outcome data precluded the development of any absolute indications for the use of flow-directed pulmonary artery catheters. Instead, the panel was forced to issue its recommendations "based on expert opinion and formed by scientific evidence." The panel stated that the pulmonary artery catheterization should be considered in surgical settings associated with an increased risk because of complications due to hemodynamic changes. The risk of hemodynamic disturbance should be assessed as a function of three interrelated variables: the health status of the patient, the type of surgical procedure, and the characteristics of the practice setting. Therefore, despite much effort and expense, the final product of this parameter contains recommendations that are vague and of limited use to the practitioner. This is an instructive example because it shows that unless data from which objective conclusions can be drawn are available, it is not possible to formulate clinically meaningful standards. In this situation, it has been suggested that the most prudent course would be to refrain from issuing any guideline at all and to merely state that the available data do not support the establishment of any firm recommendations.

Another ASA guideline deals with transfusion practice,[21] an area of concern to cardiac anesthetists because of the frequency with which they use blood products. The methodology employed in drafting this guideline was fairly rigorous, with 1417 articles retrieved and reviewed in a literature search conducted in 1994. One hundred sixty articles were selected as relevant to the topic and were then graded as to the strength of the scientific evidence in the following categories:

    I. randomized controlled trials
  II-1. nonrandomized controlled trials
  II-2. controlled observational studies
  II-3. uncontrolled observational studies
   III. descriptive studies, expert opinion

The guideline then assesses the use of red blood cells, fresh-frozen plasma, platelet and cryoprecipitate transfusions, analyzing the strength of the evidence and making recommendations in each area. For example, the recommendations for the use of red blood cells rest on available category II-2 and II-3 evidence and expert opinion. The task force concluded that

- transfusion is rarely indicated when the hemoglobin concentration is >10 g/dL and is almost always indicated when it is <6 g/dL.
- determination of whether intermediate hemoglobin concentrates (6–10 g/dL) justify or require red blood cell transfusion should be based on the patients' risk of inadequate oxygenation.
- the use of a single hemoglobin "trigger" for all patients and other approaches that fail to consider all important physiologic and surgical factors affecting oxygenation is not recommended.

The recommendation urges practitioners to consider the surgical patient's response to a decreased hemoglobin concentration. It lists a series of factors that should influence the physician's decision to transfuse, including the patient's cardiopulmonary reserve, the rate and magnitude of blood loss, oxygen consumption, and the presence of atherosclerotic disease. This guideline appears to be methodologically sound and to contain information useful to practitioners of anesthesia.

The final guideline of the ASA series relevant to cardiac anesthesia was published in 1996 in *Anesthesiology*.[20] Practice Guidelines for Perioperative Transesophageal Echocardiography was a joint effort of the ASA and the Society of Cardiovascular Anesthesiologists, which formed a task force on transesophageal echocardiography (TEE). The guidelines contain a series of sections, including an introduction, indications, complications and contra-indications, certification, credentialling, quality assurance and training, and a list of training objectives relating to developing proficiency in the use of TEE. The indications section is divided into three categories. The first are those supported by the strongest evidence or expert opinion. This evidence demonstrates that, in these procedures, TEE is frequently useful in improving clinical outcomes and is often indicated depending on individual circumstances. In this category is the intraoperative use of TEE in conditions such as valvular repair, congenital heart surgery, and repair of hypertrophic obstructive cardiomyopathy, and in unstable patients with suspected thoracic aortic aneurysms. The second are supported by weaker evidence. In these cases, TEE may be useful in improving clinical outcomes in procedures such as intraoperative assessment of cardiac aneurysm, evaluation for the removal of cardiac tumors, assessment of suspected cardiac trauma, and pulmonary embolectomy. The third indications are supported by little current scientific or expert evidence. These include the intraoperative evaluation of myocardial perfusion, coronary artery anatomy or graft patency, endocarditis during noncardiac surgery, and monitoring for emboli during orthopedic procedures. The guideline was developed by a 12-member task force that reviewed nearly 600 scientific publications relating to TEE. Given the high standard of scientific rigor used in the development of this guideline, it is useful adjunct to practitioners of cardiac anesthesia in deciding whether TEE is warranted in the care of specific patients.

Guidelines developed by the ACC cover many areas in the field of cardiology, including Guidelines for the Evaluation and Management of Heart Failure,[33] Guideline for the Management of Patients with Acute Myocardial Infarction,[35] Guidelines for the Clinical Application of Echocardiography,[36] Guidelines for Exercise Testing,[37] and one of particular value to anesthesiologists, Guidelines for Perioperative Cardiovascular Evaluation for Noncardiac Surgery.[34]

The guideline relating to perioperative evaluation contains an eight-step algorithm for the assessment of patients undergoing noncardiac surgery. Step one is determination of the urgency of the surgery. This determines the time available for further work up. The second step is to determine whether a patient has undergone coronary revascularization within the past 5 years. If a patient has undergone coronary artery surgery within this time and has had no signs of subsequent ischemia, further work up is not warranted. Step three is the inquiry as to whether the patient has had a cardiac work up in the past 2 years. If the results of the evaluation were favorable and the patient has had no symptoms in the intervening period, further work up is not warranted. Step four is the determination of whether the patient has an unstable coronary syndrome or a major risk factor, including unstable coronary disease, decompensated congestive heart failure, symptomatic arrhythmias, or severe valvular heart disease. The presence of any of these conditions merits the cancellation or delay of surgery until a full work up has been completed. Step five asks whether the patient has any intermediate clinical predictors of risk, such as a prior myocardial infarction, angina pectoris, compensated, congestive heart failure, or diabetes mellitus. Depending on the patient's functional capacity and the operative risk posed by the surgery, patients in this category may benefit from further noninvasive testing. In step six, patients with intermediate predictors of risk who have poor functional capacity or moderate functional capacity, undergoing high-risk surgery, are best served by further cardiac work up. In step seven, surgery is generally safe for patients who have neither major nor intermediate predictors of risk and who have moderate to excellent functional capacity. In step eight, the results of noninvasive testing are used to determine further preoperative management.

A section of the guideline deals with anesthetic considerations in intraoperative management. This section opines that there appears to be no one best myocardial protective anesthetic technique; thus, the selection of technique is best left to the judgment of the anesthesiologist managing the anesthetic. The guideline does indicate that failure to achieve adequate analgesia can lead to increased release of catecholamines, resulting in myocardial ischemia or infarction. The guideline advocates the importance of attention to postoperative pain management, pointing out that adequate analgesia leads to a reduction in postoperative stress and hypercoagulability. The guideline questions the use of TEE, stating that the "incremental value of this technique for risk prediction is small." In general, this guideline is a well written, helpful asset to those providing anesthesia to cardiac patients.

The Society of Thoracic Surgeons has also published an extensive set of guidelines targeted at the practitioners of thoracic and cardiovascular surgery.[23–31] The guidelines all take a common approach, that of an outline dealing with the diagnosis, procedure, indication, confirmation of indication, relative contraindications, actions before procedure, actions during procedure, actions after procedure, outcome, and references. The guidelines have been published on the following topics: ischemic heart disease;[25] valvular heart disease;[30] thoracic aortic disease;[29] chest wall, diaphragm, mediastinum, and pericardium;[23] esophageal disease;[24] bronchopulmonary disease;[26] transplantation and heart assist devices;[28] electrical problems;[31] and congenital heart disease.[27] The skeletal nature of these guidelines provides little in the way of guidance to the practitioner. For example, the guideline Ischemic Heart Disease II[25] deals with coronary atherosclerosis. The procedure advocated for the treatment of this condition is coronary artery bypass grafting (CABG). In this brief guideline, a series of 26 indications for the use of CABG surgery are listed. Confirmation that CABG is warranted is by "coronary arteriography and/or noninvasive testing as indicated." The relative contraindication is "risk judged greater than benefit." Actions advocated after the procedure include "cardiorespiratory support and treat arrhythmias." The outcomes listed include "1) one to twenty percent mortality determined by patient age and condition, associated disease, coronary anatomy, and left ventricular function; 2) discharge in less than ten days in uncomplicated cases; and 3) relief of ischemic conditions." Only two references are listed, one of which is the guideline for coronary artery bypass graft surgery published by the ACC. The effectiveness of these guidelines is hampered by a number of factors, including their terse and skeletal nature, their reliance on generalizations, and the lack of supporting references.

The AHCPR has also published a number of guidelines that are relevant to the practice of cardiac medicine. These include guidelines on cardiac rehabilitation,[98] treatment of left ventricular failure,[145] treatment of unstable angina,[97] and acute pain management in the perioperative setting.[146] The acute pain management guideline, first published in 1992, was the first guideline developed by AHCPR.[146] It was formulated using a rigorous scientific methodology and an interdisciplinary panel of experts. The guideline includes the development methodology as an appendix, as well as an extensive bibliography of the sources used. The treatment of perioperative pain is an important consideration in cardiac patients, and this guideline may contain some information useful in the care of these patients. The guidelines relating to left ventricular failure, unstable angina, and cardiac rehabilitation, similarly contain information that may be of some use to cardiac anesthesiologists, but they will not be routinely consulted. For example, the guideline on unstable angina contains the following headings: initial evaluation and treatment, outpatient care, intensive medical care, nonintensive medical care, noninvasive testing, cardiac catheterization and myocardial revascularization, hospital discharge and postdischarge care, and medical record. The section dealing with cardiac catheterization and myocardial revascularization does not contain any specific references to anesthetic management of patients undergoing CABG.[97]

CONCLUSIONS

The use of clinical practice guidelines in medicine has seen significant growth in the past 10 years. Given the extensive development that has taken place in guideline formulation in many areas of medicine, cardiac medicine included, it is somewhat surprising that there has been little work in the specific area of cardiac anesthesiology. Whether guideline development in this area will become more widespread is uncertain. When properly designed and publicized, clinical practice guidelines can be integrated into the daily practice of medicine and can result in greater standardization of care with higher quality and lower costs. On the other hand, patient management guidelines can have ill effects as well. Poorly designed guidelines based on weak evidence can deprive physicians of clinical judgment and confuse patients and caregivers alike. Practice guidelines appear to be here to stay, but much more research is needed to identify area in which guidelines can be most effective and to refine and standardize methodological techniques for guideline development. Further research must also define ways in which guidelines can be more effectively disseminated and implemented and how the effectiveness of guidelines can be assessed, both in the short- and long-term. Given the current situation, guidelines remain a tool for improving healthcare whose potential has not yet been, and perhaps never will be, fully realized.

References

1. Kelly JT, Toepp MC: Practice parameters: development, evaluation, dissemination, and implementation. QRB Qual Rev Bull 18:405,1992
2. American Medical Association. Directory of Practice Parameters. American Medical Association Office of Quality Assurance and Health Care Organizations, 1989
3. Swartout JE (ed): Directory of Practice Parameters. American Medical Association Office of Quality Assurance and Health Care Organizations, 1992
4. Walker RD, Howard MO, Lambert MD, Suchinsky R: Medical practice guidelines. West J Med 161:39, 1994
5. Field MJ, Lohr KN (eds): Guidelines for Clinical Practice: From Development to Use. Washington, DC, National Academy Press, 1992
6. Eddy DM: A Manual for Assessing Health Practices and Designing Practice Policies: The Explicit Approach. Albany, NY, ACP Press, 1992
7. American Medical Association: Attributes to Guide the Development of Practice Parameters. American Medical Association Office of Quality Assurance and Health Care Organizations, 1990
8. American Medical Association: Evaluation of practice parameters. QA Rev 3:4, 1991
9. American Medical Association: Using Practice Parameters in Quality Assessment: Quality Assurance and Quality Improvement Programs. American Medical Association, Office of Quality Assurance and Health Care Organizations, 1992
10. Hayward RSA, Wilson MC, Tunis SR: Users' guides to the medical literature. VIII. How to use clinical practice guidelines. A. Are the recommendations valid? JAMA 274:570, 1995
11. Wilson MC, Hayward RSA, Tunis SR: Users' guides to the medical literature. VIII. How to use clinical practice guidelines. B. What are the recommendations and will they help you in caring for your patients? JAMA 274:1630, 1995
12. Lomas J, Anderson GM, Domnick-Pierrek K, Vayda E, Enkin MW, Hannah WJ: Do practice guidelines guide practice? The effect of a consensus statement on the practice of physicians. N Engl J Med 321:1306, 1989
13. Mittan BS, Tonesk X, Jacobson PD: Implementing clinical practice guidelines: Social influence strategies and practitioner behavior change. QRB Qual Rev Bull 18:413, 1992
14. Woolf SH: Practice guidelines, a new reality in medicine. II. Methods of developing guidelines. Arch Intern Med 152:946, 1992
15. Woolf SH: Practice guidelines, a new reality in medicine. I. Recent developments. Arch Intern Med 150:1811, 1990

16. Battista RN, Hodge MJ: Clinical practice guidelines: Between science and art. Can Med Assoc J 148:385, 1993
17. White LJ, Ball JR: Integrating practice guidelines with financial incentives. QRB Qual Rev Bull 16:50, 1990
18. Ellrodt AG, Conner L, Riedinger MS, Weingarten S: Implementing practice guidelines through a utilization management strategy: The potential and the challenges. QRB Qual Rev Bull 18:456, 1992
19. American Society of Anesthesiologists Task Force on Pulmonary Artery Catheterization: Practice guidelines for pulmonary artery catheterization: A report by the American Society of Anesthesiologists Task Force on Pulmonary Artery Catheterization. Anesthesiology 78:380, 1993
20. American Society of Anesthesiologists and Society of Cardiovascular Anesthesiologists Task Force on Transesophageal Echocardiography: Practice guidelines for perioperative transesophageal echocardiography: A report by the American Society of Anesthesiologists and the Society of Cardiovascular Anesthesiologists Task Force on Transesophageal Echocardiography. Anesthesiology 84:986, 1996
21. American Society of Anesthesiologists Task Force on Blood Component Therapy: Practice guidelines for blood component therapy: A report by the American Society of Anesthesiologists Task Force on Blood Component Therapy. Anesthesiology 84:732–747, 1996
22. Laussen PC, Reid RW, Stene RA, Pare DS, Hickey PR, Jonas RA, Freed MD: Tracheal extubation of children in the operating room after atrial septal defect repair as part of a clinical practice guideline. Anesth Analg 82:988, 1996
23. Ferguson TB: Practice guidelines in cardiothoracic surgery: Chest wall diaphragm, mediastinum and pericardium I, II and III—A report by the Soceity of Thoracic Surgeons. Ann Thorac Surg 53:729, 1992
24. Vaneoko RM: Practice guidelines in cardiothoracic surgery: Esophageal disease I, II and III—A report by the Society of Thoracic Surgeons. Ann Thorac Surg 53:1138, 1992
25. Jones RH: Practice guidelines in cardiothoracic surgery: Ischemic heart disease I, II and III—A report by the Society of Thoracic Surgeons. Ann Thorac Surg 53:930, 1992
26. Fosberg RG: Practice guidelines in cardiothoracic surgery: Bronchopulmonary disease I-IV—A report by the Ad Hoc Committee for Cardiothoracic Surgical Practice Guidelines. Ann Thorac Surg 56:1203, 1993
27. Lindesmith GG: Practice guidelines in cardiothroacic surgery: Congenital heart disease I, II and III—A report by the Ad Hoc Committee for Cardiothoracic Surgical Practice Guidelines. Ann Thorac Surg 56:1434, 1993

28. Pennington DG: Practice guidelines in cardiothoracic surgery: Transplantation and heart assist devices I-IV—A report by the Ad Hoc Committee for Cardiothoracic Surgical Practice Guidelines. Ann Thorac Surg 58:903, 1994
29. Coselli JS: Practice guidelines in cardiothoracic surgery: Thoracic aorta disease I, II and III—A report by the Ad Hoc Committee for Cardiothoracic Surgical Practice Guidelines. Ann Thorac Surg 58:1207, 1994
30. Bartley TD: Practice guidelines in cardiothoracic surgery: Valvular heart disease I, II and III—A report by the Ad Hoc Committee for Cardiothoracic Surgical Practice Guidelines. Ann Thorac Surg 59:1264, 1995
31. Pomerantz M, Rainer WG: Practice guidelines in cardiothoracic surgery: Cardiac electrical problems I-IV—A report by the Ad Hoc Committee for Cardiothoracic Surgical Practice Guidelines. Ann Thorac Surg 59:1613, 1995
32. American College of Cardiology/American Heart Association Task Force on Practice Guidelines: Guidelines for clinical intradardiac electrophysiological and catheter ablation procedures: A report of the American College of Cardiology/American Heart Association Task Force on Practice Guidelines (Committee on Clinical Intracardiac Electrophysiologic and Catheter Ablation Procedures). J Cardiovasc Electrophysiol 6:652, 1995
33. American College of Cardiology/American Heart Association Task Force on Practice Guidelines: Guidelines for the evaluation and mangement of heart failure: A report of the American College of Cardiology/American Heart Association Task Force on Practice Guidelines (Committee on Evaluation and Management of Heart Failure). J Am Coll Cardiol 26:1376, 1995
34. American College of Cardiology/American Heart Association Task Force on Practice Guidelines: Guidelines for perioperative cardiovascular evaluation for noncardiac surgery: A report of the American College of Cardiology/American Heart Association Task Force on Practice Guidelines (Committee on Perioperative Cardiovascular Evaluation for Noncardiac Surgery). J Am Coll Cardiol 27:910, 1996
35. American College of Cardiology/American Heart Association Task Force on Practice Guidelines: Guidelines for the management of patients with acute myocardial infarction: A report of the American College of Cardiology/American Heart Association Task Force on Practice Guidelines (Committee on Management of Acute Myocardial Infarction). J Am Coll Cardiol 28:1328, 1996
36. American College of Cardiology/American Heart Association Task Force on Practice Guidelines: Guidelines for the clinical ap-

plication of echocardiography: A report of the American College of Cardiology/American Heart Association Task Force on Practice Guidelines (Committee on Clinical Application of Echocardiography). Circulation 95:1686, 1997
37. American College of Cardiology/American Heart Association Task Force on Practice Guidelines: Guidelines for exercise testing: Executive summary—A report of the American College of Cardiology/American Heart Association Task Force on Practice Guidelines (Committee on Exercise Testing). Circulation 96:345, 1997
38. Alston RP: Guidelines and cardiac anesthetists: Not in my back yard. Anaesthesia 52:328, 1997
39. Eddy DM: Practice policies: What are they? JAMA 263:877, 1990.
40. Shomaker TS: Practice policies in anesthesia: A foretaste of practice in the twenty-first century. Anesth Analg 80:388, 1995
41. Sigerist H: A History of Medicine: Primative and Archaic Medicine, p. 481, Oxford, Oxford University Press, 1951
42. Pierce EC: The development of anesthesia guidelines and standards. QRB Qual Rev Bull 16:61, 1990
43. Pierce EC: Historical perspectives. In Pierce EC, Cooper JB (eds): Analysis of Anesthetic Mishaps. International Anesthesiology Clinics. p. 22, 1984
44. Snow J: On the fatal cases of the inhalation of chloroform. Edinburgh Med Surg J 72:75, 1849
45. Lyman HM: Artificial Anaesthesia and Anaesthetics. William Wood and Company, 1881
46. American Society of Anesthesiologists: Annual Directory of Members: Guidelines for Patient Care in Anesthesiology. American Society of Anesthesiologists, 1968
47. American Society of Anesthesiologists: Annual Directory of Members: Guidelines for a Minimally Acceptable Program of Any Continuing Education Requirement. American Society of Anesthesiologists, 1989
48. American Society of Anesthesiologists: Annual Directory of Members: Guidelines for Critical Care in Anesthesiology. American Society of Anesthesiologists, 1986
49. American Society of Anesthesiologists: Annual Directory of Members: Guidelines for Delineation of Clinical Privileges in Anesthesiology. American Society of Anesthesiologists, 1989
50. American Society of Anesthesiologists: Annual Diretory of Membership: Guidelines for Ambulatory Surgery Facilities. American Society of Anesthesiologists, 1988
51. American Society of Anesthesiologists: Annual Directory of Membership: Basic Standards for Preanesthesia Care. American Society of Anesthesiologists, 1982

52. American Society of Anesthesiologists: Annual Directory of Membership: Peer Review in Anesthesiology. American Society of Anesthesiologists, 1989
53. American Society of Anesthesiologists: Annual Directory of Membership: Standards for PostAnesthesia Care. American Society of Anesthesiologists, 1990
54. Ready LB: Practice guidelines for acute pain management in the perioperative setting: A report by the American Society of Anesthesiologists Task Force on Pain Management, Acute Pain Section. Anesthesiology 82:1071, 1995
55. American Society of Anesthesiologists: Annual Directory of Members: Standards for Basic Intraoperative Monitoring. American Society of Anesthesiologists, 1993
56. Eichhorn JH, Cooper JB, Cullen DJ, Maier WR, Philip JH, Seeman RG: Standards for patient monitoring during anesthesia at Harvard Medical School. JAMA 256:1017, 1986
57. Caplan RA, Posner KL, Ward RJ, Cheney FW: Adverse respiratory events in anesthesia: A closed claims analysis. Anesthesiology 72:828, 1990
58. Tinker, JH, Dull DL, Caplan RA: Role of monitoring devices in the prevention of anesthetic mishaps: A closed claims analysis. Anesthesiology 71:541, 1989
59. Orkin FK, Cohen MM, Duncan PG: The quest for meaning in outcomes. Anesthesiology 78:417, 1993
60. Keats AS: Anesthesia mortality in perspective. Anesth Analg 71:113, 1990
61. Leape LL: Practice guidelines and standards: An overview. QRB Qual Rev Bull 16:42, 1990
62. Field MJ, Lohr KN (eds): Clinical Practice Guidelines: Directions for a New Program. Vol. 38. Washington, DC, National Academy Press, 1990
63. Carter A: Clinical practice guidelines. Can Med Assoc J 147:1649, 1992
64. Gottlieb LK, Margolis CZ, Schoenbaum SC: Clinical practice guidelines at an HMO: Development and implementation in a quality improvement model. QRB Qual Rev Bull 16:80, 1990
65. Kelly JT, Swartwout JE: Development of practice parameters by physician organizations. QRB Qual Rev Bull 16:54, 1990
66. Eddy DM: Designing a practice policy: Standards, guidelines and options. JAMA 263:3077, 1990
67. Bowsher CA: Medical Malpractice: A Continuing Problem with Far Reaching Implications. General Accounting Office, 1990
68. Pollard v Goldsmith, 117 Ariz 363, 572 P2d 1201, 1203 (Ariz Ct App 1977)

69. Bradford v McGee, 534 S2d 110 (Ala 1988)
70. James v Wooley, 523 S2d 110 (Ala 1988)
71. Holzier JF: The advent of clinical standards for professional liability. QRB Qual Res Bull 16:71, 1990
72. Evidence-Based Medicine Working Group: Evidence-based medicine: A new approach to teaching the practice of medicine. JAMA 268:2420, 1992
73. Ellrodt G, Look DJ, Lee J, Cho M, Hunt D, Weingarten S: Evidence-based disease management. JAMA 278:1687, 1997
74. Larsen RA, Evans RS, Burke JP, Pestotnick SL, Gardner RM, Classen DC: Improved perioperative antibiotic use and reduced surgical wound infections through the use of computer decision analysis. Infect Control Hosp Epidemiol 10:316, 1989
75. Tierney WM, Miller MF, Overhage JM, McDonald CJ: Physician inpatient order writing on micro computer work stations: Effects on resource utilization. JAMA 269:379, 1993
76. Cochrane AL: Effectiveness and Efficiency: Random Reflections on Health Services. Nuffield Provincial Hospitals Trust, 1972
77. Chalmers I, Dickersin K, Chalmers TC: Getting to grips with Archie Cochrane's agenda. BMJ 305:786, 1992
78. Linzer M: Critical appraisal: More work to be done. J Gen Intern Med 4:457, 1989
79. Greenspan AM, Kay HR, Berger BC: Incidents of unwarranted implantation of permanent cardiac pacemakers in a large medical population. N Engl J Med 318:158, 1988
80. Kahn KL, Kosecoff J, Soloomon DH, Brook RH: The use and misuse of upper gastrointestinal endoscopy. Ann Intern Med 109:664, 1988
81. Chassin MR, Kosecoff J, Solomon DH, Brook H: How coronary angiography is used. JAMA 258:2543, 1987
82. Winslow CM, Solomon DH, Chassin MR, Kosecoff J, Merrick NJ, Brook RH: The appropriateness of carotid endarterectomy. N Engl J Med 319:721, 1988
83. Winslow CM, Kosecoff J, Chassin MR, Kanouse DE, Brook RH: The appropriateness of performing coronary artery bypass surgery. JAMA 260:505, 1988
84. Graboys TB, Headley A, Lown B, Lampert S, Blatt CM: Results of a second opinion program for coronary artery bypass graft surgery. JAMA 258:1611, 1987
85. Kosecoff J, Kanouse DE, Brook RH: Changing practice patterns in the management of primary breast cancer: Concensus development programs. Health Serv Res 25:809, 1990
86. Appelbaum PS: Practice guidelines in psychiatry and their implications for malpractice. Hosp Community Psychiatry 43:341, 1992

87. Bulger RJ: Letter from the interest group on Health Services Research, Association of Academic Health Centers. J Qual Improvement 19:303, 1993
88. Anderson GF, Lave JR, Russe CM: Providing Hospital Services: The Changing Financial Environment. Baltimore, The John's Hopkins University Press, 1989
89. Lobach DF, Hammond WE: Computerized decision support based on a clinical practice guideline improves compliance with core standards. Am J Med 102:89, 1997
90. Browman GP, Levine MN, Mohide EA, Hayward RS, Pritchard KI, Gafni A, Laupacis A: The practice guidelines development cycle: A conceptual tool for practice guidelines development and implementation. J Clin Oncol 13:502, 1995
91. Robinson ML: Medical practice guidelines may affect payment. Hospitals 62:30, 1988
92. Zhanel GG: Affect of interventions on prescribing of antimicrobials for prophylaxis in obstetric and gynecologic surgery. Am J Hosp Pharmacol 46:2493, 1989
93. Chodoff P, Crowley K: Clinical practice guidelines: roadblocks to their acceptance and implementation. J Outcome Manage 2:5, 1995
94. Dans PE: Credibility, cookbook medicine and common sense: Guidelines the college. Ann Intern Med 120:966, 1994
95. Eddy DM: Practice policies: Guidelines for methods. JAMA 263:1839, 1990
96. Kanouse DE, Brook RH, Winkler JP, et al: Changing medical practice through technology assessment: An evaluation of the NIH Consensus Development Program. Santa Monica, CA, The RAND Corporation, 1987
97. Braunwald E, Brown J, Brown L, et al: Diagnosing and Managing Unstable Angina: Clinical Practice Guideline. United States Public Health Service, Agency for Health Care Policy and Research, 1994
98. Wegner NK, Froelicher ES, Smith LK, et al: Cardiac Rehabilitation: Clinical Practice Guideline. United States Public Health Service, Agency for Health Care Policy and Research, 1995
99. Haynes RB: Some problems in applying evidence in clinical practice. Ann N Y Acad Sci 703:210, 1993
100. Fink A, Brook RH, Kosecoff J: Sufficiency of clinical literature on the appropriate uses of six medical and surgical procedures. West J Med 47:609, 1987
101. Woolf SH, Battista RN, Anderson GM, Logan AG, Wang E: Assessing the clinical effectiveness of preventive maneuvers: Analytic principles and systematic methods in reviewing evidence and developing clinical practice recommendation. J Clin Epidemiol 43:891, 1990
102. Canadian Task Force on the Periodic Health Examination: The periodic health examination. Can Med Assoc J 121:1193, 1979

103. Cook DL, Guyatt GH, Laupacis A, Sackett PL: Rules of evidence and clinical recommendations on the use of antithrombotic agents. Chest 102(Suppl):305, 1992
104. Sackett DL: Rules of evidence in clinical recommendations on the use of antithrombotic agents. Chest 95(Suppl):2, 1989
105. Hlatky MA: Patient preferences and clinical guidelines. JAMA 273:1219, 1995
106. Agency for Health Care Policy and Research, Center for Research Dissemination and Liaison: Paper presented at the Conference on Effect Dissemination of Clinical and Health Information. Tuscon, AZ, September 22–24, 1991
107. Van Amringe M, Shannon TE: Awareness, assimilation, and adoption: The challenge of effective dissemination and the first AHCPR-sponsored guidelines. QRB Qual Res Bull 18:397, 1992
108. Haynes RB, Johnston ME, McKibbon KA, Walker CJ: A randomized controlled trial of a program to enhance clinical use of MEDLINE. Online Journal Current Clinical Trials, 1993
109. Covell DG, Uman GC, Manning PR: Information needs in office practice: Are they being met? Ann Intern Med 103:596, 1985
110. Brook RH: Practice guidelines and practicing medicine: Are they compatible? JAMA 262:3027, 1989
111. Jones L: Mixed message on mammography. Am Med News 3:1, 1993
112. American Cancer Society: Summary of Current Guidelines for Cancer Related Checkup: Recommendations. American Cancer Society, 1988
113. National Cancer Institute: Working Guidelines for Early Detection; Rationale and Supporting Evidence to Decrease Mortality. National Cancer Institute, 1987
114. American Medical Association: Mammography Screening in Asymptomatic Women 40 Years and Older: Report of the Council of Scientific Affairs. American Medical Association, 1988
115. American College of Obstetricians and Gynecologists, Committee on Professional Standards: Standards for Obstetric and Gynecological Services (6th ed). American College of Obstetricians and Gynecologists, 1985
116. American College of Radiology: Policy Statement: Guidelines for Mammography. American College of Radiology, 1982
117. Fletcher SW, Black W, Harris R: International workshop on screening for breast cancer. J Natl Cancer Inst 85:1644, 1993
118. Smigel K: NCI proposes new breast cancer screening guidelines. J Natl Cancer Inst 85:1626, 1993
119. Fram DS: A critical review of adult health maintenance. III. Prevention of cancer. J Fam Pract 22:511, 1986
120. Hayward RS, Steinberg EP, Ford DE, Roizen MF, Roach KW: Preventive care guidelines: 1991. Ann Intern Med 114:758, 1991

121. US Preventive Services Task Force: Guide to Clinical Preventive Services: An Assessment of the Effectiveness of 169 Interventions—Report of the US Preventive Services Task Force. Baltimore, Williams & Wilkins, 1989
122. Volkers N: Board recommends changes to draft breast cancer screening guidelines. J Natl Cancer Inst 85:1794, 1993
123. AHCPR, AAHP and AMA to develop national clinical guideline clearinghouse [press release]. Agency for Health Care Policy and Research, May 28, 1997
124. Lomas J, Haynes RB: A taxonomy in clinical review of tested strategies for the application of clinical practice recommendations: From "official" to "individual" clinical policy. Am J Prev Med 4:77, 1988
125. Kosecoff J, Kanouse DE, Rogers WH, McCloskey L, Winslow CM, Brook RH: Effects of the National Institutes of Health Consensus Development Program on physician practice. JAMA 258:2708, 1987
126. Tunis SR, Hayward RSA, Wilson MC, Rubin HR, Bass EB, Johnston M, Steinberg EP: Internists' attitudes about clinical practice guidelines. Ann Intern Med 120:956, 1994
127. Haines A, Feder G: Guidance on working guidelines: Writing them is easier than making them work. BMJ 305:785, 1992
128. Asaph JW, Janoff K, Wayson K, Kilberg L, Graham M: Carotid endarterectomy in a community hospital: A change in physician's practice patterns. M J Surg 161:616, 1991
129. Herman R: Harvard HMO improves pap smear screening. QA Rev 1:2, 1989
130. North of England Study of Standards and Performance in General Practice: Medical audit in general practice. II. Effects on health of patients with common childhood diseases. BMJ 304:1484, 1992
131. Russell I, Grimshaw J: The effectiveness of referral guidelines: A review of the methods and findings of published evaluations. In Roland M, Coulter A (eds): Hospital Referrals. Oxford, Oxford University Press, 1992
132. Eagle KA, Mulley AG, Skates SJ, et al: Length of stay in the intensive care unit: effects of practice guidelines and feedback. JAMA 264:992, 1990
133. Lomas J, Enkin M, Anderson GM, et al: Opinion leaders vs audit and feedback to implement practice guidelines. JAMA 265:2202, 1991
134. Schaffner W, Ray WA, Federspiel CF, Miller WO: Improving antibiotic prescribing and office practice: A controlled trial of three educational methods. JAMA 250:1728, 1983
135. Stross, JK, Bole GG: Evaluation of a continuing education program in rheumatoid arthritis. Arthritis Rheum 23:846, 1980

136. Southerai SB, Avorn J: Principles of education outreach ("academic detailing") to improve clinical decision making. JAMA 263:549, 1990
137. Spiegle JS, Shapiro MF, Berman B, Greenfield S: Changing physician test ordering in the university hospital: An intervention of physician participation, explicit criteria, and feedback. Arch Intern Med 149:549, 1989
138. Burns LR, Denton M, Goldfein S, Warrick L, Morenz B, Sales B: The use of continuous quality improvement methods in the development and dissemination of medical practice guidelines. QRB Qual Res Bull 18:434, 1992
139. Myers SA, Gleicher WA: A successful program to lower cesarian section rates. N Engl J Med 319:1511, 1989
140. Weingarten S, Erman B, Bolus R, Reidinger MS, Rubin H, Green A, Karns K, Ellrodt AG: Early "step down" transfer of low risk patients with chest pain. Ann Intern Med 113:283, 1990
141. Larsen RA, Evans RS, Burke JP, et al. Improved perioperative antibiotic use and reduced surgical wound infection through the use of computer decision analysis. Infect Control Hosp Epidemiol 10:316, 1989
142. McCullough J, Steeper TA, Connelly DP, et al: Platelet utilization in a university hospital. JAMA 259:2414, 1988
143. Lubarsky DA, Glass PSA, Ginsberg B, Dear GL, Dentz ME, Gan TJ, Sanderson IC, Mythen MG, Dufore S, Pressley CC, Gilbert WC, White WD, Alexander M, Coleman RL, Rogers M, Reeves JG: The successful implementation of pharmaceutical practice guidelines: Analysis of associated outcomes and cost savings. Anesthesiology 86:1145, 1997
144. Eichhorn JH: Prevention of intraopertive anesthesia accidents and related severe injury through safety monitoring. Anesthesiology 70:572, 1989
145. Konstam MA, Dracup K, Baker DW, et al: Heart Failure: Evaluation and Care of Patients with Left Ventricular Systemic Dysfunction—Clinical Practice Guidelines. United States Public Health Service Agency for Health Care Policy and Research, 1994
146. Carr DB, Jacox AK, Chapman CR, et al: Acute Pain Management: Operative or Medical Procedures and Trauma: Clinical Practice Guideline. US Public Health Service Agency for Health Care Policy and Research, 1992

Karen B. Domino

8 | Closed Claims Analysis as a Tool for Outcome Assessment

Adverse anesthesia outcomes are relatively infrequent events that each individual practitioner will seldom observe. Important sources for details about severe adverse outcomes are medical malpractice claims. Thus, the analysis of resolved or closed malpractice claims is a useful tool for the assessment of outcome and quality of care. However, there are a number of important limitations in the use of closed malpractice claims for outcome assessment. In this chapter, I review these limitations and illustrate the utility of malpractice claims in outcome and quality assessment using the American Society of Anesthesiologists (ASA) Closed Claims database.

LIMITATIONS OF CLOSED CLAIMS ANALYSIS

There are significant limitations with the use of malpractice claims for assessment of outcome and quality of care: they represent only a small subset of adverse outcomes, the incidence of the outcome cannot be calculated, and they contain multiple sources of bias (Table 8–1).

Subset of Adverse Outcomes

One of the most important limitations of closed claims analysis is that malpractice claims represent only a small fraction of adverse outcomes.[1–6]

Outcome Measurements, edited by Kenneth Tuman, Lippincott Williams & Wilkins, Baltimore © 1999

TABLE 8–1. LIMITATIONS OF CLOSED CLAIMS ANALYSIS

Subset of adverse outcomes
   Few adverse outcomes end in malpractice claims
   Bias toward more severe injuries
Inability to calculate incidence
   Lack of denominator data
   Geographic imbalance
Miscellaneous sources of bias
   Changes in practice patterns
   Partial reliance on direct participants
   Retrospective transcription of data
   Absence of rigorous comparison groups
   Judgment of appropriateness of care
   Poor prediction of quality of care

In the mid-1970s, at the height of the malpractice crisis, only about 10% of injuries due to provider error resulted in a malpractice claim.[1] Similar estimates were observed a decade later.[2–5] The Harvard Medical Practice study of patients hospitalized in New York in 1984 found that almost 4% of hospitalized patients sustained an iatrogenic injury, and nearly 30% of these adverse events were due to negligence. While most (70%) resulted in disability lasting <6 months, 3% of the events caused permanently disabling injuries, and 14% led to death.[3] However, only 8 of the 280 patients (<3%) who had adverse outcomes due to medical negligence filed malpractice claims.[5] The investigators estimated that, in New York, only one of eight adverse events associated with negligence resulted in a medical malpractice claim.[5] Even fewer adverse outcomes, not necessarily associated with negligence, led to malpractice claims (approximately 1 of 25 adverse events).

The relationship between malpractice claims and adverse outcomes is illustrated in Figure 8–1.[6] Area A represents all medical injuries among hospitalized patients, estimated at approximately 4% of all patient admissions.[1–5] Area B represents all errors by healthcare providers, the extent of which is unknown. Area C represents the subset of adverse patient outcomes due to error or negligence (about 1% of all hospital admissions).[3] The fraction of outcomes represented by medical malpractice claims is represented by Area D. A small percentage of adverse events due to error end in a malpractice claim, and many of the claims filed are associated with care that was judged inappropriate.[5] Area E signifies filed claims resulting in claimant compensation, estimated at about 1 in 25 patients who experience an injury.[6] Therefore, while malpractice claims provide useful information about adverse outcomes, they are comprise of a highly selective subset that may not be a representative cross-section of all adverse outcomes.

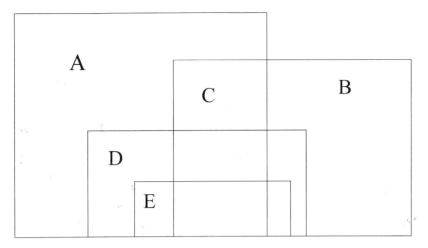

FIGURE 8–1. Relationships among adverse outcomes, errors during medical care, and malpractice claims. A, incidence of patient injuries; B, incidence of errors during medical care; C, patient injuries due to errors during medical care; D, filed malpractice claims; E, filed claims resulting in claimant compensation. Published with permission of the publisher from Goldfield N, Nash DB (eds): Providing Quality Care: The Challenges to Clinicians. © 1989, American College of Physicians, Philadelphia, PA.

There are multiple factors that influence whether an adverse outcome results in a malpractice claim, including socio-cultural factors, physician-patient interactions, the severity of the outcome, and the expected compensation for damages.[7–9] Surveys of randomly selected patients suggest that there is a large number of patients who are dissatisfied with their medical care. Twelve to twenty-five percent of adults feel that either they or a close relative have had at least one episode of harm as a result of medical treatment;[7,8] however, <10% had contacted an attorney. Patients informally consult with family members, friends, lawyers, and medical professionals to decide whether to pursue a lawsuit.[7,8] Many factors influence the patients' decisions to contact an attorney, including poor relationships with the providers, television advertisements, recommendations from healthcare providers, impressions of not being kept informed or appropriately referred by providers, and financial concerns.[9] Although calls to attorneys are frequent, few lead to a lawsuit. Only 1 in 30 calls to plaintiff law firms by patients result in the filing of a lawsuit.[9] The major reason for attorneys to decline a potential lawsuit is insufficient severity of injury and compensation for damages.[9] Attorneys generally reject claims with potentially recoverable damages of less than $50,000.[9] Therefore, analysis of closed claims is biased toward the more severe outcomes, which pay higher compensation to the plaintiff.

Inability to Calculate Incidence

There is no way to provide numerical estimates of risk because of the lack of denominator data, i.e., the number of patients undergoing anesthesia. Although some authors have attempted to relate all malpractice claims filed in a state to the number of hospital admissions,[1–5] such analyses are cumbersome and imprecise. It is even more difficult to relate these claims to the number of patients undergoing different types of anesthesia care.

In many cases, there is no control over the geographic balance in the source of claims, which depends on the organizations that allow access to the files. For instance, more than three fourths of the claims in the ASA Closed Claims database originated in the Northeast, upper Midwest, and West Coast. Relatively few claims originate in Southern states due to the lack of access to insurance company files in these states. Practice patterns and outcomes may vary regionally throughout the United States.

Miscellaneous Sources of Bias

There are several other sources of bias in the closed claims data. Cases span a period of time, during which anesthetic agents and practice patterns change. As it may take many years for a claim to be settled, analysis of closed claims frequently evaluates outcomes from old patterns of care, which may not reflect modern anesthesia practice and safety. In addition, it may take many years to detect a change in outcome with changes in practice patterns. For instance, the ASA Closed Claims Project is just now beginning to evaluate a significant number of claims in the 1990s, when new monitoring standards were universally employed.

Other limitations include the partial reliance on data from direct participants rather than impartial observers, as plaintiff and physician correspondence and depositions are the sources of information used by reviewers. Information of the outcomes is recorded retrospectively and is limited to that transcribed on a data sheet by the reviewers, who, in turn, depend on the information contained in the insurance company file. Important medical records, such as anesthesia records, may be missing from insurance company files. In addition, there is an absence of rigorous comparison groups.

There are also ambiguities in the judgment of the appropriateness of care. Appropriate or standard care has been defined as "that which met the standard for a prudent anesthesiologist practicing anywhere in the United States at the time of the event."[10] Substandard care has been defined as "that below the standard of practice (i.e., negligence)."[10] Examples of substandard care included cases in which the patient was not appropriately monitored, shortcuts in care were taken, or serious errors in judgment were made, or if there was a poor choice and/or conduct of anesthesia. The standard of care was designated as "impossible to judge" if there was not enough information in the file for the reviewer to make a judgment about standard of care.[10]

Interrater reliability is relatively low in the complex judgment of standard of care.[11,12] Anesthesiologist reviewers agreed on the standard of care in 62% of claims and disagreed in 38% of claims.[12] This bias raises several concerns about peer review and suggests that divergent opinions may be easily found among multiple experts.

The judgment of the appropriateness of care is influenced by the severity of the outcome.[13] To study this question, anesthesiologist reviewers were asked to rate the appropriateness of care in cases involving adverse outcomes. The original case involved either a temporary or permanent outcome. An alternate case identical to the original case was constructed, except that a plausible outcome of opposite severity was substituted. Examples of these cases included brain damage after airway obstruction, brachial plexus injury, seizures, eye injury, pneumothorax, ulnar nerve injury, and aspiration of gastric contents. Knowledge of the severity of injury resulted in a significant inverse effect on judgment of appropriateness of care. The proportion of ratings for appropriate care decreased by 31% when the outcome was changed from temporary to permanent and increased by 28% when the outcome was changed from permanent to temporary.[13]

Malpractice claims data have also been used as a quality improvement tools.[14,15] Malpractice claims of New Jersey physicians practicing anesthesiology, obstetrics and gynecology, general surgery, and radiology were reviewed to identify problem-prone clinical processes.[14,15] Half of the negligence claims were associated with patient management errors, such as making the wrong diagnosis, making the right diagnosis but selecting the wrong treatment, or improperly communicating treatment decisions to the patient.[14] Between one third and one half of all errors were related to improper technical performance of procedures in all specialties other than radiology.[14] Medical and nursing staff coordination resulted in only about 10% of the claims. The low incidence of improper monitoring in anesthesiology may reflect recent trends in intraoperative monitoring. The authors of that study believed that malpractice data could be used to identify systematic problems in clinical interventions and to suggest interventions that may reduce negligence. However, the authors found that using physicians' malpractice claims histories to target individuals for education or sanction is problematic because of their poor predictive power.[15] Only physician specialty was predictive of physician error profiles.[15]

ASA CLOSED CLAIMS DATABASE

Study Methodology

The ASA Closed Claims Project is a structured evaluation of adverse anesthetic outcomes obtained from the closed claim files of 35 professional liability insurance companies in the United States. One company processes claims from more than 40 states. The other sources are mainly statewide organizations that include both physician-owned and private companies. These organizations insure approximately 14,500 anesthesiologists. There are a total of 4,183 claims for adverse outcomes that originated between 1961 and 1995 in the database. Sixty-eight percent of the claims occurred between 1980 and 1990.

To collect data, one or more trained practicing anesthesiologists visited each insurance company office to review all files for claims against anesthesiologists. A standardized data collection instrument was completed for claims in which there was enough information to reconstruct the sequence of events and to determine the nature and causation of injury. The closed claim files typically consisted of relevant hospital and medical records, narrative statements from involved healthcare personnel, expert and peer reviews, deposition summaries, outcome reports, and the cost of settlement or jury award. The reviewer used standardized instructions to complete a standardized form, which records information on patient characteristics (age, sex, weight, and physical status), date of procedure, surgical procedures, anesthetic agents and techniques, monitors employed, sequence and location of events, critical incidents, clinical manifestations of injury, complications and outcomes, whether a lawsuit was filed, and the amount of the award. Reviewers assessed the overall appropriateness of anesthetic care and its contribution to the injury. They also summarized the sequence of events in each case. Each data collection focus was reviewed and approved by the three practicing anesthesiologists of the Closed Claims Study Committee in Seattle, WA.

Each claim was assigned a severity of injury score that was designated by the on-site reviewer using the insurance industry's 10-point scale. This ordinal scale rates severity of injury from 0 (no injury) to 9 (death).[10] A value of 1 represents emotional injury; 2–4 reflect temporary injuries; 5 reflects permanent, nondisabling injuries; and 6–8 reflect permanent and disabling injuries. For purposes of analysis, injuries were grouped into two categories: temporary/nondisabling (0–4) and disabling/permanent/death (5–9).

General Description

Most cases in the ASA Closed Claims database involve relatively healthy adults undergoing nonemergency surgery; 60% are female, 86% are adult (>16 years), 70% are ASA physical status I or II, 73% underwent nonemergency surgery, and 72% involve general anesthesia. Of the claims, 54% are from 1970–1984, 32% are from 1985–1989, and 14% are from the 1990s.

The claims are categorized by two factors: complications and damaging events. A complication is the injury that the patient sustained. The damaging event is the specific incident that led to the injury. The most frequent complications (Fig. 8–2) were death (32%), brain damage (12%), and nerve damage (16%). Claims for low-severity injuries account for close to 15% of the claims and include emotional distress (4%), pain during surgery (2%), awareness (2%), back pain (3%), headache (3%), and skin reaction (1%). Less frequent severe complications were the need for prolonged ventilatory support, airway trauma, eye damage, aspiration, newborn brain damage, and myocardial infarctions. The most common mechanisms of injury were respiratory system damaging events (26%), cardiovascular system damaging events (9%), misuse or failure of equipment (10%), and wrong misuse or failure of dose or drug (4%). The damaging event was not known in almost half of the cases.

Care was judged appropriate in 46% of the cases in the ASA Closed Claims database in which the appropriateness of care could be judged. The frequency of award to the plaintiff is linked to appropriateness of care but not to severity of injury.[10] An award was received in 80% of cases

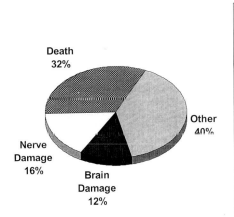

FIGURE 8–2. Complications in closed claims database (4183 claims).

in which the care was substandard, in contrast to 40% of the cases in which the standard of care was met, regardless of the severity of injury (Fig. 8–3). The magnitude of the award was linked to both severity of injury and to standard of care.[10] Nondisabling injuries were associated with lower awards than injuries that produced disabilities or death. Substandard care especially increased the award for disabling injuries, with a fivefold increase in median award (Fig. 8–4).[10] Adverse outcomes judged preventable with better monitoring were far more costly than those that were not considered preventable with better monitoring.[10] Table 8–2 illustrates the award for the most common complications in the database.

Patterns of Patient Injury

Cardiac Arrest During Spinal Anesthesia

During review of the first 900 claims, 14 cases of unexpected cardiac arrest in healthy adults were identified.[16] Each patient experienced a sudden cardiac arrest approximately 30 min after initiation of spinal anesthesia, usually preceded by stable hemodynamics and respiration. Although cardiopulmonary resuscitation was promptly initiated, epinephrine was not administered until an average of 7 min after arrest. A

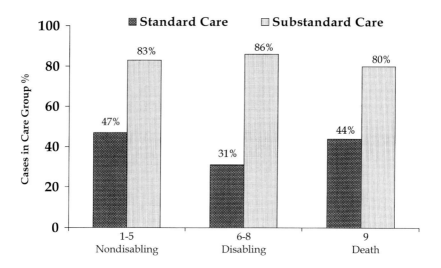

Cheney, et al.: JAMA 261:1599-1603, 1989

FIGURE 8–3. Standard of care in claims that resulted in an award to the plaintiff. Published with permission of the publisher from Cheney FW, Posner K, Caplan RA, Ward RJ: Standard of care and anesthesia liability. JAMA 261:1599–1603, 1989.

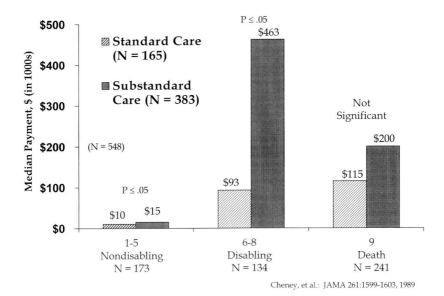

FIGURE 8–4. Median payment is influenced by the severity of injury and standard of care. Published with permission of the publisher from Cheney FW, Posner K, Caplan RA, Ward RJ: Standard of care and anesthesia liabliity. JAMA 261:1599–1603, 1989.

TABLE 8–2. PAYMENT OF MOST COMMON INJURIES ($n = 4183$)

Adverse Outcomes	Claims (%)	Median Payment ($)	Range of Payment ($)
Death	32	200,000	250–6,336,738
Nerve damage	16	35,000	157–7,600,000
Brain damage	12	687,478	2,750–23,200,000
Airway trauma	6	25,000	25–1,150,000
Emotional trauma	4	16,000	390–9,000,000
Eye damage	4	25,000	25–1,000,000
Headache	3	9,000	752–200,000
Fetal/newborn injury	4	393,285	18,248–6,800,000
Back pain	3	32,500	2,000–1,150,000
Pneumothorax	4	36,000	500–9,000,000
Aspiration	2	195,327	390–1,700,000

major factor in the poor outcome (six patients died, eight had permanent brain damage) seemed to be the inadequate appreciation of the need for early treatment of cardiac arrest with α-agonists to counteract sympathetic blockade. Recent laboratory work in dogs[17] has confirmed that total spinal anesthesia decreases coronary perfusion during cardiopulmonary resuscitation to levels below the threshold for successful resuscitation. Administration of epinephrine increases coronary perfusion above this threshold.

Review of 20 more recent cases in which pulse oximetry was used confirmed that a circulatory mechanism is most important. Although the mechanisms are unclear, vagal-linked or vagal-inducing stimuli (traction, movement, fear, pitocin, athletic heart syndrome) were frequently observed. This suggests an interaction between block of cardioaccelerator fibers by high spinal or epidural blockade and increased vagal tone.

Adverse Respiratory Events

Adverse respiratory events constitute the single largest source of injury (26% of the database) and are characterized by a high frequency of devastating and costly outcomes. A detailed analysis of these claims was published in 1990.[18] The most common mechanisms of injury were inadequate ventilation or oxygenation (7% of the entire database), difficult tracheal intubation (6%), and esophageal intubation (5%).

The proportion of respiratory-related claims has decreased with time, representing 35% of claims in the 1970s, 27% in the 1980s, and 14% in the 1990s ($P < 0.05$).[19] Preliminary data also suggest that the severity of injury is decreasing, as indicated by decreases in the proportion of claims for brain damage and death in the 1990s (Fig. 8–5).[19] The decrease in respiratory claims and severity of injury may repre-

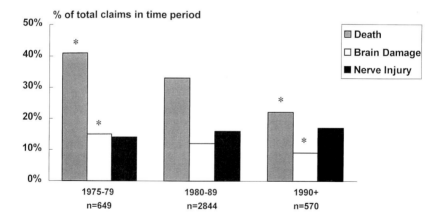

FIGURE 8–5. Most common complications by year of event. *$P \leq 0.05$ for 1975–79 versus 1990+.

sent the beneficial impact of pulse oximetry and end-tidal capnography on the diagnosis and treatment of esophageal intubation and inadequate ventilation and oxygenation. It is also unlikely that these modalities will improve outcome in cases of difficult intubation, which are becoming more common. Most cases of difficult intubation have been judged as providing appropriate care, without deficiencies in monitoring. However, as it takes 3–5 years for a claim to close, the data from the 1990s must be interpreted with caution. Therefore, data from the analysis of closed malpractice claims suggest, but do not prove, that pulse oximetry and end-tidal capnography have improved patient safety.

Pediatric Anesthesia

Ten percent of claims were in the pediatric age group (<16 years); 22% of these claims involved children <1 year of age. A review of these claims was published in 1993.[20] Injuries in pediatric claims were more severe than those in adult claims ($P < 0.01$). Of the pediatric patients, 49% died and 28% had brain damage, compared with 33% and 11% of adults, respectively. Nerve injury was relatively uncommon in the pediatric claims (2%) compared with the adult claims (17%; $P < 0.01$). The mechanism of injury in pediatric claims was more apt to be of respiratory origin (39%) compared with adult claims (25%; $P < 0.01$). Inadequate ventilation was responsible for 15% of all pediatric claims, compared with 6% of all adult claims ($P < 0.01$).

In summary, although closed claims possess a number of limitations, their analysis is useful for assessment of infrequent outcomes and quality improvement. The analysis of closed malpractice claims in the next several years will help to evaluate the impact of pulse oximetry and end-tidal capnography on adverse outcomes from anesthesia.

References

1. Danzon PM: Medical Malpractice: Theory, Evidence, and Public Policy. Harvard University Press, 1985
2. Hiatt HH, Barnes BA, Brennan TA, Laird NM, Lawthers AG, Leape LL, Localio AR, Newhouse JP, Peterson LM, Thorpe KE: A study of medical injury and medical malpractice. N Engl J Med 321:480–484, 1989
3. Brennan TA, Leape LL, Laird NM, Hebert L, Localio AR, Lawthers AG, Newhouse JP, Weiler PC, Hiatt HH: Incidence of adverse events and negligence in hospitalized patients: Results of the Harvard Medical Practice Study I. N Engl J Med 324:370–376, 1991

4. Leape LL, Brennan FA, Laird N, Lawthers AG, Localio AR, Barnes BA, Hebert L, Newhouse JP, Weiler PC, Hiatt H: The nature of adverse events in hospitalized patients: Results of the Harvard Medical Practice Study II. New Engl J Med 324:377–384, 1991
5. Localio AR, Lawthers AG, Brennan TA, Laird NM, Hebert LE, Peterson LM, Newhouse JP, Weiler PC, Hiatt HH: Relation between malpractice claims and adverse events due to negligence: Results of the Harvard Medical Practice Study III. N Engl J Med 325:245–251, 1991
6. Morlock LL, Lindgren OH, Mills DH: Medical malpractice and clinical risk management. In: Goldfield N, Nash DB (eds): Providing Quality Care: Future Challenges. 2nd ed, pp. 163–183, Health Administration Press, 1995
7. Hickson GB, Clayton EW, Githens PB, Sloan FA: Factors that prompted families to file medical malpractice claims following perinatal injuries. JAMA 267:1359–1363, 1992
8. Meyers AR: "Lumping it:" The hidden denominator of the medical malpractice crisis. Am J Public Health 77:1544–1548, 1987
9. Huycke LI, Huycke MM: Characteristics of potential plaintiffs in malpractice litigation. Ann Intern Med 120:792–798, 1994
10. Cheney FW, Posner K, Caplan RA, Ward RJ: Standard of care and anesthesia liability. JAMA 261:1599–1603, 1989
11. Posner KL, Sampson PD, Caplan RA, Ward RJ, Cheney FW: Measuring interrater reliability among multiple raters: An example of methods for nominal data. Stat Med 9:1103–1115, 1990 [published erratum appears in Stat Med 11:1401, 1992]
12. Posner KL, Caplan RA, Cheney FW: Variation in expert opinion in medical malpractice review. Anesthesiology 85:1049–1054, 1996
13. Caplan RA, Posner KL, Cheney FW: Effect of outcome on physician judgments of appropriateness of care. JAMA 265:1957–1960, 1991
14. Kravitz RL, Rolph JE, McGuigan K: Malpractice claims data as a quality improvement tool. I. Epidemiology of error in four specialties. JAMA 266:2087–2092, 1991
15. Rolph JE, Kravitz RL, McGuigan K: Malpractice claims data as a quality improvement tool. II. Is targeting effective? JAMA 266:2093–2097, 1991
16. Caplan RA, Ward RJ, Posner K, Cheney FW: Unexpected cardiac arrest during spinal anesthesia: A closed claims analysis of predisposing factors. Anesthesiology 68:5–11, 1988
17. Rosenberg JM, Wahr JA, Sung CH, Oh YS, Gilligan LJ: Coronary perfusion pressure during cardiopulmonary resuscitation after spinal anesthesia. Anesth Analg 82:84–87, 1996
18. Caplan RA, Posner KL, Cheney FW: Adverse respiratory events in

anesthesia: A closed claims analysis. Anesthesiology 72:828–833, 1990
19. Cheney FW: Anesthesia patient safety and professional liability continue to improve. ASA Newsletter 61:18–20, 1997
20. Morray JP, Geiduschek JM, Caplan RA, Posner KL, Gild WM, Cheney FW: A comparison of pediatric and adult closed malpractice claims. Anesthesiology 78:461–67, 1993.

Index

Page references followed by *t* or *f* indicate tables or figures, respectively.

β-Adrenergic blockers
   effects on cardiovascular outcomes after noncardiac surgery, 107–115
   perioperative use in noncardiac surgical patients at risk from coronary artery disease
      guidelines for, 115–120
      protocol for, 120, 121*f*
      trial of, 107–115
Adverse occurrence rate, as measure of quality of care, 7–15
Adverse respiratory events, closed malpractice claims related to, 168*f*, 168–169
Agency for Healthcare Policy Research, practice guidelines
   development of, 135–137
   dissemination of, 138
   relevant to cardiac medicine, 146–147
American College of Cardiology and American Heart Association, practice guidelines, 126, 129–130
   practice guidelines, affecting cardiac anesthesia, 145–146
American College of Physicians, guidelines for assessing and managing perioperative risk from coronary artery disease in noncardiac surgery, 115–119
American Society of Anesthesiologists
   Guidelines for Patient Care in Anesthesiology, 128
   practice guidelines, and cardiac anesthesia, 141–145
   practice standards and guidelines, 128–130
American Society of Anesthesiologists Closed Claim Study, 50. *See also* Closed claims analysis
   cases in
     of adverse respiratory events, 168*f*, 168–169
     awards in, 166, 166*f*–167*f*, 167*t*
     of cardiac arrest during spinal anesthesia, 166–168
     characteristics of, 165*f*–167*f*, 165–166, 167*t*
     patterns of patient injury in, 166–169
     pediatric anesthesia-related, 169
   methodology for, 164
Angina, unstable, definition of, 83
Angioplasty, outcomes assessment, data for, 73–76, 74*t*, 75*f*, 75*t*
Atenolol
   and cardiovascular outcomes after noncardiac surgery, 107–115
   perioperative use in noncardiac surgical patients at risk from coronary artery disease, 107–115
      guidelines for, 115–120
      protocol for, 120, 121*f*
Atenolol trial, 107–115
   adverse effects and side effects of atenolol in, 114–115, 117*t*
   and cardiovascular medication use before and after surgery, 114, 116*t*
   clinical implications of, 115
   drug administration in, 108–109
   findings in, 109–115

Atenolol trial—*Continued*
  indicators of treatment effect in, 109–115
  long-term results of, 111t, 111–112, 112f–114f
  mortality in
    early, 112, 113f, 114
    overall, 111–112, 114f
    predictors of, 113–114, 115t
  patient selection for, 107–108
  rationale for, 107
  survival after
    in diabetics, 113–114, 115t
    event-free, 112, 113f
    overall, 111t, 111–112, 113f
  tolerance of atenolol in, administration route and, 114–115, 117t

BARI. *See* Bypass Angioplasty Revascularization Investigation
Bayes' theorem, 89–92
Beta-blockers. *See* β-Adrenergic blockers
Bias
  in administrative data, 88
  in case-control studies, 87
  in closed claims analysis
    miscellaneous sources of, 162–164
    toward severe outcomes, 159–161, 161f
  control of, randomized clinical trials and, 27, 48
  in data used in meta-analysis, 33–34
  in observational data, 50–51
  in outcomes research on quality of care, 15–19
  referral, 95–97
β-Blockers. *See* β-Adrenergic blockers
Breast cancer
  outcome prediction in, 88
  screening, guidelines for, 139–140
  trials, fraud in, 27
Bypass Angioplasty Revascularization Investigation, 74–76, 75f, 75t

Cardiac arrest during spinal anesthesia, closed malpractice claims related to, 166–168

Cardiac morbidity and mortality, perioperative, in noncardiac surgical patients
  cost of, 105
  incidence of, 105
Cardiac Risk Index, 84, 85t, 94
Cardiac Surgery Reporting System, assessment of, 15t, 15–16
Cardiovascular outcome(s)
  after noncardiac surgery
    β-adrenergic blockers and, 107–115
    factors affecting, 105–107
    and healthcare costs, 105
    and management of high-risk patients, 115–120, 121f
    morbidity and mortality related to, 105
  definition of, 82–83
Care. *See also* Healthcare
  access to, practice guidelines and, 132
  appropriateness of
    analysis of, 40–41, 41f, 44
    judgment of, 162–163
  quality of. *See* Quality of care
  standards of. *See* Standards of care
  substandard, 162–163
  value-based comparisons of, 44–46, 46t
Carotid endarterectomy
  appropriateness of care analysis for, 40–41
  outcomes, hospital-specific improvement efforts, 56
  small-area variation analysis for, 42–44, 43f
Case-controlled studies
  bias in, 87
  principles and rationale for, 86–87
Charlson Index of Comorbidities, 88
Clinical database(s)
  current issues related to, 76–78
  data collection for, 77
  data quality and, 77–78
  focus of, 68
  form of, 68–69
  function of, 68
  statistical methods and, 78
Clinical decision making. *See also* Decision analysis
  improvement of, application of outcomes research for, 54–60, 55f

Clinical information system
  current issues related to, 76–78
  data collection for, 77
  data quality and, 77–78
  specifications for, 67–69
  statistical methods and, 78
Clinical practice guidelines. *See* Practice guidelines
Clinical prediction rule, 58. *See also* Outcome prediction
Clinical trials. *See also* Randomized clinical trials
  statistical analysis of, problems with, 36
Closed claims analysis. *See also* American Society of Anesthesiologists Closed Claim Study
  bias in
    miscellaneous sources of, 162–164
    toward severe outcomes, 159–161, 161*f*
  limitations of, 159–164, 160*t*
Cohort studies
  in perioperative risk stratification, 95–98
  prospective, 84–85, 85*t*
Comorbidity, analysis of, 88–89
Complication rates, as measure of quality of care, 3–5, 7–15
Congestive heart failure, definition of, 83
Construct validity
  definition of, 3
  of outcomes measure, 3–5
Cooperative Cardiovascular Project, 71*f*, 71–72, 72*f*
Coronary artery bypass grafting
  appropriateness of care analysis for, 40–41
  outcomes
    assessment, data for, 73–76, 74*t*, 75*f*, 75*t*
    hospital-specific improvement efforts, 56
    variations, reduction of, 55–56
  small-area variation analysis for, 42*f*, 42–44
  transfusion practice for, 56
Coronary artery disease
  and cardiovascular outcomes after noncardiac surgery
    in atenolol trial, 107–115

  factors affecting, 105–107
  and healthcare costs, 105
  morbidity and mortality related to, 105–107
  outcome prediction in patients with, principles of, 81–100
  perioperative risk from, in noncardiac surgery, guidelines for assessment and management of, 115–120
  risk factors for, 107–108
  testing for, 89–92
Coronary revascularization, before noncardiac surgery, decision analysis on value of, 98*f*, 98–100, 99*f*
Cost containment, practice guidelines and, 132, 134
Cost-effectiveness analysis, use and misuse of, 44–46
Costs. *See also* Healthcare costs
  hospital charges as surrogate marker for, 26
Cost-savings
  outcomes and, 59
  practice guidelines and, 31, 59
Critical care outcomes, variations in, reduction of, 56–57

Data analysis, 92–95
Database(s)
  administrative, 69, 87–89
    analysis, in cardiovascular research, 72*f*, 72–73, 73*f*–74*f*, 87–88
    strengths and weaknesses of, 88–89
  clinical. *See* Clinical database
  large
    cardiovascular research using, 69–76, 87–89
    observational studies using, 29–32, 50, 69–70
  observational, evaluation of, 70
  population, 69
  in quality assurance, 71
  retrospective, outcomes analysis using, 29–32
  secondary, observational studies using, 50–51
Data torturing, 36
Death rates, as measure of quality of care, 3–5, 7–15

Decision analysis
  definition of, 98
  on value of preoperative testing and potential interventions, 98f, 98–100, 99f
Decision tree, definition of, 98
Diagnostic test(s)
  predictive value of, 89, 90t, 91f, 91–92, 92f, 97
  preoperative
    decision analyses on value of, 98f, 98–100, 99f
    in perioperative risk stratification, 96–98
  sensitivity of, 89, 90t
  specificity of, 89, 90t
Disease registries, 69
Duke Databank for Cardiovascular Disease, 74–76, 75f, 75t
Dysrhythmia(s), perioperative, in atenolol trial, 110, 110t

Economic evaluation, of healthcare outcomes and technology, 54
Effectiveness, versus efficacy, 70
Efficacy, versus effectiveness, 70
Electrocardiography, ST-segment changes, 83
Error, type II (β), 94
Evidence-based medicine
  application of, problems with, 139
  practice guidelines and, 131, 139

Failure to rescue, as outcome measure, 7–15
Framingham Heart Study, 84

Global Utilization of Streptokinase and TPA (Alteplase) for Occluded Coronary Arteries database, 76, 76t
Goldman Cardiac Risk Index. *See* Cardiac Risk index

Healthcare. *See also* Care
  appropriateness of, analysis of, 40–41, 41f, 44
  improvement of, application of outcomes research for, 54–60, 55f
  value-based, 40
  variation in, reduction of, 55–57

Healthcare costs. *See also* Cost-savings
  marketplace responses to, 46–47
  and practice guidelines, 131–132, 134
  and quality of care, 40–44
Healthcare delivery, small-area variation in, 42f, 42–44, 43f, 55
Heart rate
  intraoperative, in atenolol trial, 109, 109t
  postoperative increase in, 106–107
Hemodynamics, intraoperative, in atenolol trial, 109, 109t
High-risk patients, outcomes for, 30, 56
Hospital charges, as surrogate marker for costs, 26

Inflammation, and perioperative cardiac morbidity and mortality, 106

Malpractice claims. *See also* Closed claims analysis
  as quality improvement tools, 163–164
  as subset of adverse outcomes, 159–161, 161f
Malpractice liability, practice guidelines and, 132
Managed care, 131–132
Medicare database, analysis of, in cardiovascular research, 72f, 72–73, 73f–74f, 87–88
Meta-analysis
  in cardiovascular research, 94–95
  and cohort trials, 95
  pros and cons of, 33–34
  and randomized clinical trials, 34, 95, 96f
  rationale for, 32–33, 95
Multivariate analysis, 93t, 94
Myocardial infarct/infarction
  diagnostic criteria for, 82–83
  outcomes
    analysis of, 71f, 71–73, 72f–74f
    hospital-specific improvement efforts, 56
  postoperative, outcome measure for, 25
  prognosis for, 82–83

Myocardial ischemia
  definition of, 83
  immediate postoperative, in emergence from anesthesia, 106
  perioperative, in atenolol trial, 110, 110t
  postoperative
    factors associated with, 106
    medical therapy for, 106–107
    pharmacologic prophylaxis of, 106–107

National Institutes of Health (NIH), Consensus Development Program, 135
Nausea and vomiting, postoperative, outcome measure for, 25–26
Noncardiac surgery
  cardiac morbidity and mortality in patients undergoing
    cost of, 105
    incidence of, 105
  cardiovascular outcomes after
    β-blockers and, 107–115
    factors affecting, 105–107
    and management of high-risk patients, 115–120, 121f
  coronary revascularization before, decision analysis on value of, 98f, 98–100, 99f
  in patients at risk from coronary artery disease
    guidelines for assessing and managing, 115–119
    perioperative β-blocker therapy and, 115–120
  patients undergoing, algorithm for assessment of, 145
  perioperative cardiac complications of, 105
Northern New England Cardiovascular Disease Study Group, results, assessment of, 16–19

Observational studies, problems with, 29–32, 50–52
Outcome(s)
  assessment of, data for, 73–76, 74t, 75f, 75t
  cardiovascular. See Cardiovascular outcome(s)
  clinical, 52–53, 53t
  definition of, 52
  economic consequences as, 53t, 54
  functional health status as, 53, 53t
  patient-related, 53t
  patient satisfaction as, 53t, 54
  prediction, in coronary artery disease, 58, 81–100
    issues related to perioperative period, 95–98
  variation in, reduction of, 55–57
Outcome measure(s)
  construct validity of, 3–5
  and correction for severity of illness, 2–3
  definitions of outcome, uniformity of, 6
  failure to rescue as, 7–15
  ideal, properties of, 2t, 2–6
  observed outcomes using, uniformity of, 6
  in outcomes research, 52–54, 53t
  predictability of, 2
  recording of outcomes using, uniformity of, 6
  as reflection of quality of care, 2
  selection of, 24–27
  statistical power of, 5t, 5–6
  surrogate, 52–53
  use of, 24–27
Outcomes research
  application of, to improvement of care, 54–60, 55f
  conventional clinical research and, comparison of, 49, 49t, 51–52
  definition of, 47–48
  development of, 40–47
  as effectiveness research, 49
  outcomes in, 52–54, 53t
  on quality of care, 15–19

Pain management, practice guidelines for, 142–143, 146
Parameters, 130
Patient empowerment, practice guidelines and, 132
Patient preferences, for care, research possibilities for, 59–60
Patient satisfaction, as outcome, 53t, 54
Pediatric anesthesia, closed malpractice claims in, 169
Pharmaceutical practice guidelines, cost-savings and outcomes with, 31, 59

Power analysis, 23–24, 34–36
Practice guidelines
  advantages and disadvantages of, 132–134
  affecting cardiac anesthesia, 141–147
  British cardiac anesthetists' position on, 126–127
  for cardiac care, 141–147
  definition of, 129
  departures from, 129–130
  development of, 125–126, 134–138
    methodology for, 134–138
  dissemination of, 138
  effectiveness of, 141
    criteria for evaluation of, 134
  and healthcare costs, 131–132, 134
  historical perspective on, 127–129
  implementation of, 139–140
  integration into medical practice, 140, 147
  national clearinghouse on, 140
  need for, 131–134
  and outcomes, 31
  for pain management, 142–143
  principles and rationale for, 125–126
  relevant to cardiovascular anesthesia, 126–127
  role in 21st-century healthcare, 132
  and standards of care, comparison of, 130–131
Practice policies, 129–130
Practice standards, 130
Process measurement, 70–73
Production function, 44, 45f
Professional autonomy, practice guidelines and, 132
Prospective cohort studies, 84–85
Protocols, 129–130
Pulmonary artery catheter/catheterization
  appropriate use in CABG, clinical prediction rule for, 58
  case-controlled study of, 87
  practice guidelines for, 143
  selective use of, 57–58

Quality assurance
  databases in, 71
  practice guidelines and, 132

Quality of care
  assessment of, outcomes analysis in, 1–20
  complication rates as measure of, 3–5, 7–15
  and healthcare costs, 40–44
  outcomes research on, 15–19

Randomized clinical trials, 27–32
  blinded, 27, 85
  and meta-analysis, comparison of, 34
  and observational studies, comparison of, 29–32, 70
  principles and rationale for, 85–86
  single-center versus multicenter, 27–29
  strengths and weaknesses of, 48–49, 70, 86
  tight versus loose control of, 29
Retrospective studies. *See also* Case-controlled studies
  using large databases, 29–32
Risk adjustment, 51, 88
Risk assessment
  in cardiovascular disease, 51, 81–100
  preoperative testing in, Bayesian approach to, 89–92
  statistical analyses in, 92–95
Risk factors
  biological significance of, 95
  clinical significance of, 92–95
  statistical significance of, 92–95
Risk stratification, preoperative
  Bayesian approach to, 89–92
  generalizability of, 95–98
  limitations of, 95–98

Sample size, determination of, 23–24, 24t, 34–36
Society of Thoracic Surgeons, practice guidelines, 129, 146
Spinal anesthesia, cardiac arrest during, closed malpractice claims related to, 166–168
Standards of care, 130
  judgment of, interrater reliability in, 163
Statistical analysis
  discriminative, 94
  linear regression techniques, 94
  logistic regression techniques, 94

multivariate, 93t, 94
Statistical methods, and clinical information systems, 78
Statistical significance (P value), 92
Statistical test(s), 92, 93t
Study design, 25
SUPPORT Trial, 87
Surgery
    excitotoxic response to, and perioperative cardiac morbidity and mortality, 106
    noncardiac. See Noncardiac surgery
Surrogate outcome, use of, 24–27

Technology, selective use of, 57–58

Test(s)
    diagnostic. See Diagnostic test(s)
    statistical. See Statistical test(s)
Transesophageal echocardiography, perioperative, practice guidelines for, 144–146
Transfusion practice
    for coronary artery bypass grafting, 56
    practice guidelines for, 143–144
Troponin, cardiac, 83

Upcoding bias, in outcomes research on quality of care, 15–19

Value-based care, 40